Commercial Production of Monoclonal Antibodies

Bioprocess Technology

Series Editor

W. Courtney McGregor

Xoma Corporation
Berkeley, California

Additional Volumes in Preparation

Commercial Production of Monoclonal Antibodies

A Guide for Scale-Up

edited by

SALLY S. SEAVER

Hygeia Sciences
Newton, Massachusetts

MARCEL DEKKER, INC.   **New York and Basel**

Library of Congress Cataloging-in-Publication Data

Commercial production of monoclonal antibodies.

  (Bioprocess technology ; v. 2)
  Includes bibliographies and index.
  1. Antibodies, Monoclonal--Industrial applications.
2. Antibodies, Monoclonal--Synthesis. 3. Biochemical
engineering. I. Seaver, Sally S. II. Series.
TP248.M65C66 1987   615'.37   87-13631
ISBN 0-8247-7765-4

MARCEL DEKKER, INC.
270 Madison Avenue, New York, New York 10016

Current printing (last digit):
10 9 8 7 6 5 4 3 2 1

PRINTED IN THE UNITED STATES OF AMERICA

Series Introduction

The revolutionary developments in recombinant DNA and hybridoma technologies that began in the mid-1970s have helped to spawn several hundred new business enterprises. Not all these companies are aimed at producing gene products or cell products, as such. Many are supportive in nature; that is, they provide contract research, processing equipment, and various other services in support of companies that actually produce cell products. With time, some small companies will probably drop out or be absorbed by larger, more established firms. Others will mature and manufacture their own product lines. As this evolution takes place, an explosive synergism among the various industries and the universities will result in the conversion of laboratory science into industrial processing. Such a movement, necessarily profit driven, will result in many benefits to humanity.

New bioprocessing techniques will be developed and more conventional ones will be revised because of the influence of the new biotechnology. As bioprocess technology evolves, there will be a need to provide substantive documentation of the developments for those who follow the field. It is expected that the technologies will continue to develop rapidly, just as the life sciences have developed rapidly over the past 10–15 years. No single book could cover all of these developments adequately. Indeed, any single book will be in need of replacement or revision every few years. Therefore, our continuing series in this rapidly moving field will document the growth of bioprocess technology as it happens.

The numerous cell products already in the marketplace, and the others expected to arrive, in most cases come from three types of bioreactors:

(a) classical fermentation; (b) cell culture technology; and (c) enzyme bio-reactors. Common to the production of all cell products or cell product analogs will be bioprocess control, downstream processing (recovery and purification), and bioproduct finishing and formulation. These major branches of bioprocess technology will be represented by cornerstone books, even though they may not appear first. Other subbranches will appear, and over time, the bioprocess technology "tree" will take shape and continue growing by natural selection.

W. Courtney McGregor

Preface

The commercial production of monoclonal antibodies for any purpose involves much more than culturing large batches of hybridoma cells or injecting huge numbers of mice. It involves much preproduction work to ensure that the original hybridoma line is stable, not contaminated by murine viruses or *Mycoplasma*, and produces adequate amounts of antibody that is itself stable and has the desired specificity and affinity for its antigen. If not, the hybridoma line must be subcloned to select one that possesses these properties. If contaminated by viruses, the line is unsuitable for production. The commercial production of monoclonal antibodies involves building a suitable facility for the production, purification, qualification, and storage of the antibody. The facility must satisfy Good Manufacturing Procedures if the antibody is used in an FDA-controlled product. The antibody must be purified in high yield, harmful contaminants removed, and the antibody stored so that it maintains its activity—all of which depend on its final use and product claims. Effective testing of each lot is necessary to ensure the reproducibility of the product and the procedures. Finally, if the product is FDA-controlled or part of an FDA-controlled product, each step of production for each lot must be documented.

This book addresses several key aspects involved in scaling-up the production of monoclonal antibody from hybridoma cells. It is not inclusive of all that one needs to know about large-scale production. It represents the efforts of those people in industry who had the hard data on the production or purification of monoclonal antibody, the time, and the permission of their current companies to write their chapters. Each chapter emphasizes a slightly different aspect of commercial production, from tests to be done before production to new ways to monitor production, from practical problems with setting up GMP production to developing algorithms for operating reactors, from studies on hybridoma media usage to new techniques for purifying antibody. Since it is a snapshot taken in 1986 of a quickly evolving field, the book emphasizes the approaches used to solve the many issues encountered in large-scale production. The details of several techniques and other useful information are outlined separately in the appendixes at the end of the book.

This book stresses that the traditional chemical engineering approach to scale-up—producing more cells—is only part of the answer. Antibody secretion can be uncoupled from hybridoma cell proliferation. As such, what is learned from the culture of hybridoma cells, the cells with the most large-scale experience, is useful for optimizing the production of other proteins from other eukaryotic cell lines.

It is apparent on reading this book that, despite the obvious prejudices of several authors, there is no "best" system for producing or purifying monoclonal antibody. Nor will the reader discover a low-cost system for producing and purifying antibody. There are several reasons for this. First, most of the systems described can easily produce the quantities currently needed, 1-100 g. Today, it is more important to have a reliable production method than to have the least-expensive method. The cost of producing the monoclonal antibody is only a fraction of the total cost of a diagnostic kit. Therapeutic monoclonal antibodies are also price-insensitive because they are so new that there is no competition.

Second, it is impossible to determine the true costs of the various production methods. The productivity claims for each commercial system are made with very high-producing, but different strains. The intrinsic antibody secretion rate of each hybridoma cell line is genetically controlled and can vary 100-fold among hybridoma lines produced from the fusion of the same mouse strain to the same myeloma line. The productivity of a hybridoma line can usually be increased 2–10-fold in a well-designed and -operated culture system; however, the exact increase is cell line dependent. In addition, many culture systems are designed to produce partially purified and concentrated antibody, often at the expense of maintaining high cell productivity. This was a distinct advantage initially. It is much less of one since the development of methods to adapt cell lines to serum-free medium, the development of rapid methods to concentrate culture supernatant, and the development of purification procedures that selectively bind antibody.

Third, much work remains to be done on developing that low-cost system. New types of culture systems, most of them perfusion based, that increase the rate of antibody secretion per cell have been developed. Low-protein-containing, serum-free medium that reduces production costs and simplifies purification has been developed. Manufacturers have started to develop simple, rapid purification procedures for their culture systems. However, all these advances have to be integrated and automated to develop the low-cost system. This will involve determining which parameters need to be monitored and when to adequately control production. New probes that measure these critical parameters, including antibody levels, automatically and on-line, need to be developed. Effective algorithms need to be written to control the monitoring and to use the results of the monitoring to maintain the complete production system in its optimal state. In other words, the commercial production of monoclonal antibodies, or any other biological, today requires too much manual labor by people with too much education.

Be that as it may, the commercial production of monoclonal antibodies has come a long way since its inception in the early 1980s. The various aspects of the production of antibody that are discussed in this book do contain valuable information useful for anyone in industry or academia who is scaling-up the production of monoclonal antibody. You are invited to read and to apply all that is useful to your own work.

I would like to thank the individual chapter authors, who spent many hours, often after work, on writing and editing their chapters to make them clearer and easier to read. I would also like to thank those who started to write chapters but did not finish them because of changes in employers or job assignments or the withdrawal of company permission to publish. This book was written by people in industry, for whom, unlike those in academia, publication is not a primary responsibility. Their willingness to share their data and experiences is a real benefit for everyone who is producing a biological product from mammalian cells.

Sally S. Seaver

Contents

Contributors

S. Robert Adamson   Genetics Institute, Cambridge, Massachusetts 02138

Bradley G. Andersen   Endotronics, Inc., Coon Rapids, Minnesota 55433

Leo A. Behie   Department of Chemical Engineering, University of Calgary, Calgary, Alberta, Canada T2N 1N4

Timothy L. Brooks   Bio-Rad Laboratories, Richmond, California 94804

Bruce L. Brown   Hazleton Biotechnologies Company, Vienna, Virginia 22180

Joseph P. Chandler[a]   Charles River Biotechnical Services, Inc., Wilmington, Massachusetts 01887

G. Maurice Gaucher   Division of Biochemistry, Department of Chemistry, University of Calgary, Calgary, Alberta, Canada T2N 1N4

M. Judith Gemski   Waters Chromatography Division, Millipore Corporation, Fairfax, Virginia 22030

Jean M. George[b]   Damon Biotech, Needham Heights, Massachusetts 02194

Present affiliations:
[a]Ventrex Laboratories, Inc., Portland, Maine 04103.
[b]Simmons College, Boston, Massachusetts 02115.

Micheal L. Gruenberg   Endotronics, Inc., Coon Rapids, Minnesota 55433

Hector Juarez-Salinas   Bio-Rad Laboratories, Richmond, California 94804

Michael S. Kallelis[a]   Damon Biotech, Needham Heights, Massachusetts 02194

William B. Lebherz III   Program Resources, Inc., National Cancer Institute–Frederick Cancer Research Facility, National Institutes of Health, Frederick, Maryland 21701

Shwu-Maan Lee[b]   Program Resources, Inc., National Cancer Institute–Frederick Cancer Research Facility, National Institutes of Health, Frederick, Maryland 21701

Barry H. Lesser   Division of Biochemistry, Department of Chemistry, University of Calgary, Calgary, Alberta, Canada T2N 1N4

David R. Nau   J. T. Baker Chemical Company, Phillipsburg, New Jersey 08865

Gary S. Ott[c]   Bio-Rad Laboratories, Richmond, California 94804

Robert E. Peters[d]   University of California at San Diego, San Diego, California 92121

Elizabeth G. Posillico[e]   Damon Biotech, Needham Heights, Massachusetts 02194

James E. Putnam   Lilly Research Laboratories, A Division of Eli Lilly and Company, Indianapolis, Indiana 46285

Sally S. Seaver   Hygeia Sciences, Newton, Massachusetts 02160

William R. Shek   Charles River Laboratories, Inc., Wilmington, Massachusetts 01887

Present affiliations:
[a]Milligen Division, Millipore Corporation, Bedford, Massachusetts 01730.
[b]Genex Corporation, Gaithersburg, Maryland 20877.
[c]Chiron Corporation, Emeryville, California 94608.
[d]Cytotech, Inc., San Diego, California 92121.
[e]Genzyme Corporation, Boston, Massachusetts 02111.

Larry Stanker   Lawrence Livermore National Laboratory, Livermore, California 94550

M. Patricia Strickler   Waters Chromatography Division, Millipore Corporation, Fairfax, Virginia 22030

Randall J. von Wedel[a]   Bio-Response, Inc., Hayward, California 94545

---

[a]*Present affiliation*: CytoCulture International, Inc., San Francisco, California 94122.

Commercial Production of
Monoclonal Antibodies

I
BEFORE SCALING-UP PRODUCTION

1

Detection of Murine Viruses in Biological Materials by the Mouse Antibody Production Test

WILLIAM R. SHEK
Charles River Laboratories, Inc., Wilmington, Massachusetts

I. INTRODUCTION

Murine viral contaminants of biological materials have been shown to mislead researchers and invalidate experimental findings. In fact, many indigenous viruses of mice were first discovered as contaminants that altered research results (1–4). More important than virus-mediated effects on experimental responses are the dangers that murine viruses pose to the health of laboratory animals and humans (5–8). Adventitious exposures to these viruses can occur via natural routes or as a consequence of either accidental or intentional parenteral inoculation of contaminated biological materials. With the growth of the biotechnology industry, intentional parenteral inoculation of humans with murine monoclonal antibody (MAb)-based products for diagnostic and therapeutic purposes is becoming more frequent. To be used safely for these purposes, as well as to comply with government regulations (9), MAb products must be demonstrated to be free of contamination with infectious murine viruses.

To detect infectious viruses, in general, a specimen is first inoculated into a susceptible host system such as cell culture, embryonated eggs, or laboratory animals. Several approaches can then be used to demonstrate viral infection of the host (10). At various times postinoculation the host can be examined for changes characteristically associated with viral infection. These include cytopathic effects (CPE) in cell culture, pock formation and embryo death in ovo and pathologic changes, clinical signs, and mortality in laboratory

3

animals. Signs of viral infection however, may be subtle or inapparent and usually do not suffice for identification of the isolated agent.

In addition to examination of the host for virus-induced changes, cells, tissues, and fluids from the host can be tested to demonstrate the presence of virus or viral constituents. Some of the methods used to do this are electron microscopy, hemagglutination, serologic immunoassays, and nucleic acid hybridization. These methods ascertain the morphologic, antigenic, and genetic characteristics of viruses and therefore are a key component in the identification of viral isolates.

When laboratory animals are the host system, serum samples from con-valescent animals can be assayed for virus-specific antibodies formed as part of the immune response to infection. Detection of antibodies to a virus is tantamount to demonstrating previous infection of the host with that virus. This is the basis of the mouse antibody production (MAP) test for detection of murine viruses in biological materials, which will be discussed in this chapter.

The MAP test was first developed by Rowe and co-workers for the quanti-tation and detection of polyoma virus (11). Subsequently, they (2,4) and other investigators (12–14) used the MAP test to detect additional murine viruses. In a recent report to manufacturers of monoclonal antibody products for use in humans (9), the Chairman of the Food and Drug Administration's Hybridoma Committee recommended that hybridomas and the monoclonal antibodies they produce be screened for murine viral contaminants using the MAP test. Hybridoma cell lines accessioned by Charles River Biotechnical Services are routinely MAP-tested before being inoculated into mice for large-scale production of MAb.

II. MAP TEST PROCEDURE

The following is a general description of the customary MAP test procedure, based on that reported by Collins and Parker (14). Mice 4 weeks of age or older are inoculated with the specimen being MAP-tested. Viruses in the specimen cause the mice to mount an antiviral immune response. Virus-specific antibodies, produced as part of this response, are detected by serologic tests performed on serum samples collected approximately 4 weeks post-inoculation. To produce meaningful results, the MAP mice must not have been exposed to any exogenous murine viruses prior to inoculation. During the test period, MAP mice are maintained in sterilized microisolation units and manipulated in a biological safety cabinet to preclude infection with viruses other than those in the test specimen. In addition, MAP mice have to be capable of developing detectable levels of antibodies in response to each of the viral agents included in the MAP test, with the exception of lactate-dehydro-genase-elevating virus (to be discussed below). The ability to do so is principally determined by the genetic background (15, 16) and age (17) of the mice. The immune system of suckling mice is not fully developed and therefore they are much less responsive to viruses than older mice. For this reason, MAP mice are at least 4 weeks of age when inoculated.

Although noninfectious virus can be immunogenic, much higher antibody titers develop in animals following an active infection (18, 19). It follows that the likelihood of detecting viruses in a MAP specimen is greatest if they are infectious. The infectivity of virus is affected by the conditions of storage. While most viruses are stable at $-70°C$, many rapidly become noninfectious when held at $-20°C$. Some viruses are inactivated by low pH (20). We have had virus inocula in nonairtight vials become inactivated when temporarily stored on dry ice because a drastic drop in pH occurred when CO_2 from the ice dissolved in the inocula. Consequently, to preserve viral infectivity, MAP specimens are stored and shipped at or below $-65°C$ in hermetically sealed vials such as cryotubes.

The infectivity of viruses for animals is also affected by the route of inoculation. Sendai virus, being a respiratory pathogen of rodents, replicates primarily in the respiratory tract. Parker and Reynolds (12) found that MAP titers following intranasal inoculation of Sendai virus were much higher than those following intraperitoneal inoculation. To ensure optimal sensitivity, specimens are typically inoculated into MAP mice by multiple routes: intraperitoneally (IP), intranasally (IN), orally/per os (PO), and/or intracranially (IC) (14).

Besides being contingent upon the use of virus-free immunocompetent mice, meaningful results can only be achieved in the MAP test if the serologic assays for detection of viral antibodies are both sensitive and specific.

Traditionally, rodent serologic testing for viral antibodies has been done using conventional tests such as complement fixation and hemagglutination inhibition (21–23). During the past decade, however, conventional tests have been supplanted by more sensitive nonradioisotopic solid phase immunoassays including the enzyme-linked immunosorbent assay (ELISA) (reviewed in 24) and the indirect immunofluorescence assay (IFA) (25–28).

In addition to serologic testing for virus-specific antibodies, immunity to lymphocytic choriomeningitis virus (LCMV) is demonstrated by challenging specimen-inoculated mice, at or after 2 weeks postinoculation, with an IC injection of LCMV. Death between 6 and 8 days following IC challenge indicates that LCMV was not isolated from the specimen. Survival, on the other hand, indicates that the mice developed immunity in response to LCMV contamination of the specimen. It is interesting that both susceptibility and resistance to IC challenge are mediated by the cellular immune response (29). The redundancy of tests performed to detect LCMV is warranted because LCMV is a zoonotic agent reported to cause disease in humans ranging from a

Table 1 CRBS MAP Test Protocol

Inoculation[a] group	Sample	DPI collected[b]	No. of mice[c] per group	Procedure	Positive result
I/II	Serum	4–10	1	LDH	8–10-fold increase in LDH activity above normal
	Serum	≥28	4	Serology	Detection of virus-specific antibodies
	Mouse	≥14	1	IC challenge w/1000 LD of LCMV	Survival until 10 days post-challenge
Control	Serum	4–10	2	LDH	—
	Serum	≥28	2	Serology	—

[a]Each mouse is inoculated with 0.5 ml IP, 0.05 ml IN, and 0.05 ml PO of inoculum. Inoculum I is a low dilution of the specimen, II is a 10-fold dilution of I in balanced salt solution (BSS), and the control inoculum is the BSS diluent.
[b]Days postinoculation that the serum was collected.
[c]CD-1 Swiss albino mice 4–6 weeks of age and free of antibodies to the agents listed in Table 2 at the time of inoculation.

Table 2   Virus-Specific Antibodies Detected in the MAP Test

Virus	Virus group	Test Primary	Test Alternative
Sendai (SEN)	Parainfluenza	ELISA	HAI
Pneumonia virus of mice (PVM)	Paramyxo	ELISA	HAI, IFA
Mouse hepatitis virus (MHV)	Corona	ELISA	IFA
Minute virus of mice (MVM)	Parvo	ELISA	HAI, IFA
Mouse polio virus (GD-7)	Picorna	ELISA	HAI
Type 3 reovirus (Reo-3)	Reo	ELISA	HAI, IFA
Epizootic diarrhea of infant mice (EDIM)	Rota	ELISA	IFA
Mouse pneumonitis (K) virus	Papova	HAI	CF
Ectromelia (Ectro)	Pox	ELISA	IFA
Polyoma virus (Poly)	Papova	HAI	IFA
Mouse adenovirus (MAD)	Adeno	ELISA	IFA, CF
Lymphocytic choriomeningitis virus (LCMV)	Arena	ELISA	IFA
Mouse cytomegalovirus (MCMV)	Herpes	ELISA	IFA

ELISA, enzyme-linked immunosorbent assay; HAI, hemagglutination inhibition; CF, complement fixation; IFA, indirect immunofluorescence assay.

flu-like sickness to, in rare instances, fatal illness with central nervous system or hemorrhagic manifestations (5-8). In addition, LCMV infection of rodents (6,17,29) and cell lines if often not apparent (14,30).

As part of the MAP test, plasma or serum samples from specimen-inoculated mice, usually collected between 3 and 5 days postinoculation (DPI), are assayed for the level of lactate dehydrogenase (LDH) activity. Normal LDH levels are between 200 and 400 IU/L. Mice infected with lactate-dehydrogenase-elevating virus (LDV), however, have serum levels of LDH 8-10-fold higher than normal (31).

In the Charles River MAP test procedure either gnotobiotic or viral antibody-free, noninbred, CD-1 (Swiss albino) mice, 4-6 weeks of age are inoculated by multiple routes with two dilutions of the MAP specimen (Table 1). Serum samples collected no sooner than 28 DPI are tested for antibodies to the viral agents shown in Table 2. Samples that give positive or nonspecific

Table 3   MAP Test on Murine Viral Inocula

Inoculum	Origin[a]	No. of mice tested	No. positive[b]		
			SEN	PVM	MHV
SEN[c]	ATCC	3	3	0	0
PVM	ATCC	1	0	1	0
MHV-1	MCI	4	0	0	4
MHV-JHM	NCI	4	0	0	4
MHV-S	NCI	4	0	0	4
MVM	NCI	4	0	0	0
GD-7	NCI	4	0	0	0
Reo-3	NCI	4	0	0	0
K	ATCC	4	0	0	0
Vaccinia	ATCC	4	0	0	0
Poly	ATCC	4	0	0	0
MAD-FL	MA	4	0	0	0
MAD-K87	Yale	4	0	0	0
LCMV	ATCC	5	0	0	0
MCMV	ATCC	4	0	0	0

[a]ATCC, American Type Culture Collection (Rockville, Maryland); NCI, National Cancer Institute (Bethesda, Maryland); MA, Microbiological Associates (Bethesda, Maryland); Yale, Yale University Department of Comparative Medicine (New Haven, Connecticut).
[b]By primary or alternative assay in Table 2.
[c]Abbreviations for viruses defined in Table 2.
[d]Not tested.
[e]Only against MAD-K87.

				No. positive[b]				
MVM	GD-7	Reo-3	K	ECTRO	POLY	MAD	LCMV	MCMV
0	0	0	0	0	0	0	0	NT[d]
0	0	0	0	0	0	0	0	NT
0	0	0	0	0	0	0	0	0
0	0	0	0	0	0	0	0	0
0	0	0	0	0	0	0	0	0
4	0	0	0	0	0	0	0	NT
0	4	0	0	0	0	0	0	NT
0	0	4	0	0	0	0	0	NT
0	0	0	4	0	0	0	0	NT
0	0	0	0	3	0	0	0	NT
0	0	0	0	0	4	0	0	NT
0	0	0	0	0	0	4	0	NT
0	0	0	0	0	0	4[e]	0	NT
0	0	0	0	0	0	0	5	NT
0	0	0	0	0	0	0	0	4

reactions are retested by an alternate assay. MAP tests, performed at Charles River on a variety of murine viral inocula, demonstrate the immunocompetence of CD-1 mice and the specificity of the serologic assays (Table 3).

III. DETECTION OF VIRAL CONTAMINANTS BY THE MAP TESTS

Collins and Parker found that 69% of murine leukemia virus preparations and transplantable tumor tested positive on the MAP test. The contamination rate for in vitro cultures was lower than that for animal-passaged material. LDV, which causes a latent persistent infection of mice, and minute virus of mice (MVM), which has a predilection for rapidly dividing cells such as transplantable tumors, were found to be the predominant contaminants. The high incidence of adventitious viruses in animal-passaged material, according to Collins and Parker, was, at least in part, a reflection of the prevalence of viral infections in mouse colonies (22). Nettleton and Rweyemamu (32) found that fetal bovine serum was the source of a parvovirus serologically related to MVM that infected their BHK-21 cells.

Table 4   Murine Viruses Detected in Hybridoma Cell Lines and Other Biological Specimens by the MAP Test

Specimen type	No. of sources	No. of test specimens	No. positive (%)	Virus (No. positive)
Mouse hybridomas	24	77	6 (7.8)	Reo-3 (3), MHV (3)
Mouse tumor lines	7	58	30 (51.7)	LDV (20), POLY (9), MVM (2), MHV (2)
Rat tumor lines	2	11	0	—
Hamster tumor lines	1	13	3 (23.1)	LCMV (3)
Human tumor lines	3	17	0	—
Mouse serum/ascites/ MAb products	3	16	1 (6.3)	MHV (1)
Totals:		192	40	

Assays included: LDH levels, antibodies to SEND, PVM, Reo-3, MHV, MVM, GD-VII, ECTRO, LCMV, MAD, K, POLY.
Abbreviations for viruses defined in Table 2.

In MAP tests performed at Charles River (Table 4), viruses were detected in only 7.8% of 77 hybridoma cells. The viruses demonstrated were Reo-3 and MHV. The virus detection rate in nonhybridoma mouse tumor lines was 51.7%. Similarly to that reported by Collins and Parker (14), the predominant virus detected was LDV followed by polyoma, MVM, and mouse hepatitis virus (MHV). No murine viruses were found in rat or human tumor lines, but 3 of 13 hamster tumor lines were shown to contain LCMV. Virus was demonstrated in mouse serum, but not in ascites or MAb product specimens.

The low level of murine viral contaminants in hybridomas probably occurs because most of the processes involved in the production of hybridomas are carried out in vitro. Furthermore, advances in isolator and barrier technology have increased the availability and therefore the use of mice free from infection with murine viral pathogens.

IV. DECONTAMINATION OF HYBRIDOMA LINES

As is the case for cell lines contaminated with fungi, bacteria, or mycoplasma, it is best to dispose of hybridomas contaminated with murine viruses. Without question, cells containing LCMV should be immediately sterilized and disposed of in a safe manner. However, because hybridoma lines can be extremely valuable and difficult to produce, it is worthwhile to consider ways by which they might be decontaminated. The author could find no published methods.

Detection of virus in a suspension of hybridoma cells does not necessarily indicate that the cells are infected. Viruses reported to infect mouse lymphocytes and that therefore could infect hybridomas, are MHV (33), MVM (34), Reo-3 (33), Ectromelia (35), polyoma (36), LCMV (17,29), mouse cytomegalovirus (37), and mouse thymic virus (3). Any attempt to treat virus-infected cells will most probably be unsuccessful, principally because virus replication is dependent upon the metabolism of the host cells. Consequently, most treatments that are virostatic are also cytotoxic (35). Immunologic approaches to decontamination, such as incubation in vitro with macrophages (38), cytolysis with virus-specific antibody and complement, or inoculation into immune mice, in addition to being inherently cytotoxic, are ineffective against latently infected cells or when viral cell-surface antigens are not expressed. Collins and Parker (14) observed that viral contamination of some cell lines persisted even after 50 animal passages.

If hybridoma cells are not infected with the viral contaminants, decontamination by dilution of the virus during in vitro passage may be successful. LDV does not multiply in tumor cell lines and in species other than the mouse. Consequently, Plagemann and Swim (39) were able to decontaminate mouse tumor cell lines of LDV by passages in vitro or in other rodent species. Similarly, Rowe et al. (4) were able to free Moloney leukemia virus of LDV during propagation in culture.

V. COMPARISON OF THE MAP TEST TO OTHER METHODS FOR DETECTING INFECTIOUS MURINE VIRUSES

The MAP test has been compared to virus detection by inoculation of suckling mice and by isolation in cell culture. In the MAP test, inoculation of a single host system (the mouse), is sufficient for demonstrating 14 mouse viruses. By contrast, no cell culture is susceptible to all these viruses. In fact, no reliable cell culture systems yet exist for the isolation and propagation of mouse pneumonitis (K) virus, LDV, or epizootic diarrhea of infant mice (EDIM). Cell culture results can be lost because of specimen cytoxicity, bacterial and fungal contamination, or nonspecific degeneration of host cells, which problems usually do not affect the MAP test (4).

With the MAP test, virus detection and identification are simultaneous, whereas viruses detected by the other methods are usually identified only after further testing (13). However, viral agents detected in the MAP test are not isolated and hence cannot be further characterized. In addition, only currently known viruses for which there are reliable serologic assays can be demonstrated. Inoculation of a specimen into cell culture or suckling mice, on the other hand, may reveal previously unknown viruses or those not routinely demonstrated using serologic assays (4,13). Examples of the latter are mouse thymic virus, a herpes virus that causes thymic necrosis in neonatal mice (3); and murine leukemia viruses, which are demonstrated by isolation in cell culture (40–42).

The relative sensitivity of the MAP is virus-dependent. For detection of polyoma virus, Rowe et al. (11) found the MAP test to be equivalent in sensitivity to virus isolation in mouse embryo culture. Hartley and Rowe (2) subsequently showed that the MAP test gave higher titration endpoints for the FL strain of mouse adenovirus than those observed in mouse embryo cultures and suckling mice. Similarly, MAP test titration endpoints for Reo-3 and LCMV (13) and for Sendai virus (12) were reported to be comparable to endpoints in suckling mice and cell culture, respectively. Conversely, MAP titers for K virus (4) and the GD-7 strain of mouse encephalomyelitis virus (13) were substantially lower than those determined by suckling mouse inoculation.

VI. CONCLUSION

Monitoring of biological materials for viral contamination is important if we are to avoid spurious experimental findings and the wasting of valuable research resources and is essential to safeguard the health of humans and animals exposed to these materials. Monitoring should be done routinely because there are many potential sources of unwanted viruses and because infection of laboratory animals and cell cultures with these viruses is sometimes not apparent.

The MAP test is an immunologically based method for simultaneous detection and identification of murine viral contaminants in hybridomas, MAb products, and other biological specimens; it is sensitive, specific, and comprehensive. These characteristics of the MAP test are a consequence of using mice, a highly susceptible natural host, and sensitive and specific serologic assays for detecting viral antibodies.

The principal drawback of the MAP test is that it can be used only to demonstrate known viruses for which there are reliable serologic assays. In addition, comparative studies have shown that, for detection of certain murine viruses, the MAP test is less sensitive than inoculation of suckling mice. The authors of these studies (4,13) concluded that, for maximum sensitivity, the MAP test should be augmented by other methods of virus detection.

REFERENCES

1. Riley, V., Lilly, F., Huerto, E., and Bardell, D. (1960). Transmissible agent associated with 26 types of experimental mouse neoplasms. *Science* *132*:545–547.
2. Hartley, J. W. and Rowe, W. P. (1960). A new mouse virus apparently related to the adenovirus group. *Virology 11*:645–649.
3. Rowe, W. P. and Capps, W. I. (1961). A new mouse virus causing necrosis of the thymus in newborn mice. *J. Exp. Med. 113*:831–844.
4. Rowe, W. P., Hartley, J. W., and Huebner, R. J. (1962). Polyoma and other indigenous mouse viruses. In *The Problems of Laboratory Animal Disease.* Edited by R. J. C. Harris. New York, Academic Press, pp. 131–142.
5. Lewis, A. M., Rowe, W. P., Turner, H. C., and Huebner, R. J. (1965). Lymphocytic-choriomeningitis-virus in hamster tumor: Spread to hamsters and humans. *Science 150*:363–364.
6. Baum, S. G., Lewis, A. M., Rowe, W. P., and Huebner, R. J. (1966). Epidemic nonmeningitic lymphocytic-choriomeningitis-virus infection. An outbreak in a population of laboratory personnel. *N. Engl. J. Med. 274*:934–936.

14   Shek

7. Biggar, R. J., Schmidt, T. J., and Woodall, J. P. (1977). Lymphocytic choriomeningitis in laboratory personnel exposed to hamsters inadvertently infected with LCM virus. *J. Am. Vet. Med. Assoc. 171*:829–832.
8. Lehmann-Grube, F. (1981). Lymphocytic choriomeningitis. In *International Textbook of Medicine, Vol. II*, Medical Microbiology and Infectious Diseases. Edited by A. I. Braude. Philadelphia, Saunders, pp. 1254–1258.
9. Merchant, B. (1983). Points to consider in the manufacture of monoclonal antibody products for human use. Office of Biologics, FDA, July 25.
10. Hawkes, R. A. (1979). General principles underlying laboratory diagnosis of viral infections. In *Diagnostic Procedures for Viral, Rickettsial and Chlamydial Infections, 5th edition.* Edited by E. H. Lennette and N. J. Schmidt. American Public Health Association, pp. 3–48.
11. Rowe, W. P., Hartley, J. W., Estes, J. D., and Huebner, R. J. (1959). Studies on mouse polyoma virus infection. I. Procedures for quantitation and detection of virus. *J. Exp. Med. 109*:379–391.
12. Parker J. C. and Reynolds, R. K. (1968). Natural history of Sendai virus infection in mice. *Am. J. Epidemiol. 88*:112–125.
13. Lewis, V. J. and Clayton, D. M. (1971). An evaluation of the mouse antibody production test for detecting three murine viruses. *Lab Anim. Sci. 21*:203–205.
14. Collins, M. J. and Parker, J. C. (1972). Murine virus contaminants of leukemia viruses and transplantable tumors. *J. Natl. Cancer Inst. 49*:1139–1143.
15. Zinkernagel, R. M. and Doherty, P. C. (1977). Major transplantation antigens, viruses and specificity of surveillance T cells. *Contemp. Topics Immunobiology 7*:179–220.
16. Brownstein, D. G. (1983). Genetics of natural resistance to Sendai virus infection in mice. *Infect. Immun. 41*:308–312.
17. Cole, G. A. and Nathanson, N. (1974). Lymphocytic choriomeningitis pathogenesis. *Prog. Med. Virol. 18*:94–110.
18. Amerding, D., Rossiter, H., Ghazzouli, I., and Liehl, E. (1982). Evaluation of live and inactivated influenza A virus vaccines in a mouse model. *J. Infect. Dis. 145*:320–330.
19. Appel, M. J. G., Shek, W. R., Shesberadaran, H., and Norrby, E. (1984). Measles virus and inactivated canine distemper virus induce incomplete immunity to canine distemper. *Arch. Virol. 82*:73–82.
20. Fenner, F. and White, D. O. (1970). *Medical Virology.* New York, Academic Press.
21. Parker, J. C., Tennant, R. W., Ward, T. G., and Rowe, W. P. (1965). Virus studies with germfree mice. 1. Preparation of serologic diagnostic reagents and survey of germfree and monocontaminated mice for indigenous murine viruses. *J. Natl. Cancer Inst. 34*:371–380.
22. Parker, J. C., Tennant, R. W., and Ward, T. G. (1966). Prevalence of viruses in mouse colonies. In *Viruses of Laboratory Rodents.* Edited by R. Holdenried. NCI Monograph 20, U.S. Government Printing Office, pp. 25–36.

23. Descoteaux, J. P., Grignon-Archambault, D., and Lussier, G. (1977). Serologic study on the prevalence of murine viruses in five Canadian mouse colonies. *Lab Anim. Sci. 27*:621–626.

24. Parker, J. C. (1983). ELISA: An introduction. *Lab Anim. 12*:15–17.

25. Anderson, C. A., Murphy, J. C., and Fox, J. G. (1983). Evaluation of murine cytomegalovirus antibody detection by serological techniques. *J. Clin. Microb. 18*:753–758.

26. Smith, A. L. (1983). Response of weanling random-bred mice to inoculation with minute virus of mice. *Lab Anim. Sci. 33*:37–39.

27. Smith, A. L. (1983). An immunofluorescence test for detection of serum antibody to rodent coronaviruses. *Lab Anim. Sci. 33*:157–160.

28. Smith, A. L., Knudson, D. L., Sheridan, J. F., and Paturzo, F. X. (1983). Detection of antibody to epizootic diarrhea of infant mice (EDIM) virus. *Lab Anim. Sci. 33*:442–445.

29. Lehmann-Grube, F. (1982). Lymphocytic choriomeningitis virus. In *The Mouse in Biomedical Research*, Vol. II. Edited by H. L. Foster, J. D. Small, and J. G. Fox. New York, Academic Press, pp. 231–266.

30. Simon, M., Domok, I., and Pinter, A. (1982). Lymphocytic choriomeningitis (LCM) virus carrier cell cultures. *Acta Microbiol. Acad. Sci. Hung. 29*: 201–208.

31. Notkins, A. L. and Shochat, S. J. (1963). Studies on the multiplication and the properties of lactate dehydrogenase agent. *J. Exp. Med. 117*:735–747.

32. Nettleton, P. F. and Rweyemamu, M. M. (1980). The association of calf serum with contamination of BHK-21 Clone 13 suspension cells by a parvovirus serologically related to minute virus of mice (MVM). *Arch. Virol. 64*:359–374.

33. Kraft, L. M. (1982). Viral diseases of the digestive tract. In *The Mouse in Biomedical Research*, Vol. II, Diseases. Edited by H. L. Foster, J. D. Small, and J. G. Fox. New York, Academic Press, pp. 159–191.

34. McMaster, G. K., Beard, P., Engers, H. D., and Hirt, B. (1981). Characterization of an immunosuppressive parvovirus related to minute virus of mice. *J. Virol. 38*:317–326.

35. Fenner, F. (1982). Mousepox. In *The Mouse in Biomedical Research*, Vol. II. Diseases. Edited by H. L. Foster, J. D. Small, and J. Fox. New York, Academic Press, pp. 209–230.

36. Rabson, A. S. and Legallais, F. Y. (1959). Cytopathogenic affect produced by polyomavirus in cultures of milk-adapted murine lymphoma cells (strain P388D). *Proc. Soc. Exp. Biol. Med. 100*:229–233.

37. Loh, L. and Hudson, J. B. (1979). Interaction of murine cytomegalovirus with separated populations of spleen cells. *Infect. Immun. 26*:853–860.

38. Triglia, T. and Burns, G. F. A method for in vitro clearance of mycoplasma for human cell lines. *J. Immunol. Methods 64*:133–139.

39. Plagemann, P. G. W. and Swim, H. E. (1966). Relationship between the lactate dehydrogenase-elevating virus and transplantable murine tumors. *Proc. Soc. Exp. Biol. Med. 121*:1142–1146.

40. Rowe, W. P., Pugh, W. E., and Hartley, J. W. (1970). Plaque assay techniques for murine leukemia virus. *Virology 42*:1136–1139.

41. Hartley, J. W., Wolford, N. K., Old, L. J., and Rowe, W. P. (1977). A new class of murine leukemia virus associated with development of spontaneous lymphomas. *Proc. Natl. Acad. Sci. 74*:789–792.
42. Peebles, P. T. (1975). An in vitro focus-induction assay for xenotropic murine leukemia virus, feline leukemia virus C and the feline primate viruses RD-114/CCC/M-7. *Virology 67*:288–291.

2

Metabolism of Hybridoma Cells in Suspension Culture: Evaluation of Three Commercially Available Media

S. ROBERT ADAMSON
Genetics Institute, Cambridge, Massachusetts

LEO A. BEHIE, G. MAURICE GAUCHER, and BARRY H. LESSER
University of Calgary, Calgary, Alberta, Canada

I. INTRODUCTION

Monoclonal antibody (1,2) may be obtained from culture supernatants of hybridoma cells grown in vitro or from ascitic fluids produced when cells are grown in the peritoneal cavity of histocompatible rodents. Briefly, the major advantages of cell culture over ascites production of monoclonal antibody are: higher reproducibility, absence of extraneous antibody, low risk of contamination of antibody by adventitious agents of rodents, and low cost for production of large quantities of antibody. Accordingly, we are interested in increasing the efficiency of monoclonal antibody production from hybridoma cells cultured in vitro (3).

In this chapter we evaluate three commercially available growth media for their abilities to support growth of and monoclonal antibody production by hybridoma cells grown in suspension culture. These media are RPMI 1640, Dulbecco's modified Eagle medium with high glucose (DMEM), and a further modification of DMEM in which glucose has been replaced by fructose (HGEM) (4) (see below). We have determined growth and antibody production kinetics as well as maximum cell density and antibody titers attainable in these three media in the presence of conventional levels of serum and other supplements. In addition, we have monitored changes in the levels of key nutrients and waste products, and growth and antibody yields relative to the metabolites utilized. Delineating these general characteristics will ultimately allow us to tailor a medium suitable for economical, high-density culture of hybridoma cells, and, in the short term, to use commercially available growth media more efficiently.

II. MATERIALS AND METHODS

A. Materials

Mouse hybridoma cells producing monoclonal antibody to human transferrin (anti-HT cells) were a gift from Dr. T. Pearson, Department of Microbiology and Biochemistry, University of Victoria, Victoria, British Columbia, Canada. The parental myeloma cell line used was SP2/0-Ag14 (5) and the immunized spleen was obtained from a BALB/c mouse. Tests were made for the presence of mycoplasma by both a direct agar culture and an indirect staining procedure using Hoechst 33258. Assays were carried out in the laboratory of Dr. P. A. Quinn, Hospital for Sick Children, Toronto, Ontario, Canada. The materials used in enzyme-linked immunosorbent assays (ELISA) were as described previously (3). All enzymes used in enzymatic analysis were supplied by Sigma. Unless otherwise indicated, all media components were supplied by Gibco. Sulfosalycyclic acid was purchased from Pierce (catalogue number 27800). The remaining biochemicals used were of the best available reagent grade.

B. Analytical Procedures

1. pH Measurement

Measurements of pH were carried out on cell suspensions (5-10 ml) immediately (within 10 sec) after removal from spinner flasks using a pH meter with a standard glass electrode. The pH meter was standardized against phosphate buffer of known pH (Fisher Gram Pac, pH 7.41 at 25°C) at 37°C.

2. Cell Enumeration

Cell density and viability were determined using a hemocytometer after cell suspensions were stained with trypan blue.

3. Enzyme-Linked Immunoadsorbent Assay

The anti-HT antibody titers of cell-free medium were determined by ELISA as previously described (3).

4. Metabolite Assays

Ammonium was assayed in nondeproteinized, cell-free culture medium by the method of Weatherburn (6). Typically, the medium to be assayed was diluted 10-fold with deionized water and 0.5 ml diluted medium, or an appropriate dilution of an ammonium chloride standard solution, was added to 3 ml of reagent A (1 g of phenol and 5 mg sodium nitroprusside in 100 ml deionized water) and 3 ml reagent B (0.5 g sodium hydroxide and 0.8 ml sodium hypochlorite in 100 ml deionized water). The mixture was incubated at $37°C$ for 20 min, cooled to room temperature (for 5 min), and the absorbance at 625 nm was read.

Under these conditions the standard curve was linear between 0 to 4.5 μg ammonium and was unaffected by the addition of aliquots (equal to the volume of sample under assay) of the original, unconditioned medium. This control was carried out in order to take into account any possible interference in the assay by medium components.

Some reported enzyme assays for ammonia (7) are more sensitive than the previous assay. However, the latter is convenient, requires relatively small quantities of sample (50 μl), and the sensitivity of the assay is adequate (as described, the assay is accurate down to about 0.2 mM ammonium in culture medium). Furthermore, unlike enzymatic determinations, this assay does not require the samples to be deproteinized before ammonium determinations. In fact, during validation of the assay, it was observed that deproteinization (by perchloric acid, described below) caused consistently low values to be obtained.

In order to carry out assays on the remaining metabolites, samples of cell free culture medium were routinely deproteinized with perchloric acid at $0°C$ (final concentration 3%). After immediate neutralization with 1 M NaOH, the protein-free supernatant was analyzed for glucose and lactate (3), pyruvate (8), fructose (9), and glutamine plus glutamate (10) by standard enzymatic methods except that recommended assay volumes were reduced to approximately 1 ml. Concentrations of glutamine alone were calculated by subtracting the levels of glutamate, measured by conventional amino acid analysis (described below) from the additive concentrations of glutamine and glutamate measured by enzymatic analysis.

5. Amino Acid Analysis

Quantities of amino acids in aliquots of culture supernatants were determined by two different methods of automatic amino acid analysis after deproteinization by two different techniques.

Conventional Amino Acid Analysis: To 1-2 ml of cell free culture medium was added 100 μl of 5.3 mM norleucine, followed by 5 ml cold 95% ethanol

(67% final). Samples were stored overnight at 5°C and the following day the resulting precipitate was removed by centrifugation at 12,000 X g at 5°C. Ethanol was removed by evaporation in vacuo and 5 ml deionized water was added back. The samples were lyophilized and the resulting powder taken up in 150 μl of the first buffer used in amino acid analysis. Usually 50 μl of this was analyzed. Lyophilization was necessary to concentrate the sample and remove bicarbonate, which was seen to interfere with amino acid analysis. Samples were analyzed on a Beckman 121 automatic amino acid analyzer by the method of Spackman et al. (11). The original concentration of amino acids was calculated relative to the norleucine internal standard. Generally recovery, based on norleucine yield, was between 70 and 90%.

Physiological Amino Acid Analysis: Serine, threonine, glutamine, and asparagine are not easily resolved on conventional amino acid analysis, as described above. Accordingly these amino acids, in addition to hydroxy-proline and aspartic acid, were quantitated by physiological amino acid analysis on a D500 automated amino acid analyzer (Durrum). In these experiments 0.54 mL cell-free culture medium was deproteinized on ice by the addition of 50 μl of 43% sulfosalicylic acid (3.9% final concentration) (12). After a 5 min incubation on ice the precipitate was removed by centrifugation in a Beckman microfuges for 15 min at 4°C. The pH of the protein free supernatant was adjusted by the addition of 25 μl of a 2.28% solution of lithium hydroxide. Forty microliters of a suitable dilution (usually one-fifth) was analyzed. Since no concentration step was involved and considerably less sample was loaded in this method it was not necessary to remove bicarbonate.

The preferred method of analysis is the physiological system, which allows quantitation of all common and some secondary amino acids in a single analysis. Disadvantages of both the previous procedures were (a) that samples required pretreatment in order to deproteinize them and (b) the analysis was time-consuming; conventional analyses took 3 hr and physiological 3.5 hr per analysis. This problem can be improved if contemporary equipment is available; the Beckman 6300 automatic amino acid analyzer carries out conventional and physiological amino acid analysis in 30 min and 120 min, respectively. Furthermore a very rapid (30 min) method of amino acid analysis that does not require deproteinization and allows resolution of all common amino acids including glutamine, asparagine, serine, and threonine (but not cysteine or the secondary amino acids proline or hydroxyproline) has been reported recently using a high-performance liquid chromatography system employing orthophthalaldehyde precolumn derivatization (13, Appendix 4, this book).

III. EFFECTS OF MEDIA AND COMPONENTS ON HYBRIDOMA GROWTH AND ANTIBODY PRODUCTION

A. Growth and Antibody Production

In the three media tested anti-HT hybridoma cells grew during exponential growth (between days 1 and 2 of culture) with a doubling time (td ± standard error) of 15.0 ± 1.4 hr, 12.7 ± 2.0 hr, and 14.0 ± 1.5 hr to maximum cell densities (± SE) of 1.4 ± 0.2 × 10^6, 2.9 ± 0.1 × 10^6, and 1.8 ± 0.2 × 10^6 cells/ml in RPMI, DMEM, and HGEM respectively (Fig. 1). Antibody production essentially paralleled growth in all media. Only in HGEM did antibody accumulation continue after cell growth had ceased such that a maximum titer (± SE) of 2200 ± 200 was attained after 104 hr. On cessation of growth in RPMI at 69 hr an antibody titer (± SE) of 3700 ± 300 was attained. Similarly, in DMEM after growth cessation at 93 hr a titer of 2600 ± 100 had accumulated. Antibody productivities (change in titer/10^3 cells/day ± SE) during exponential growth were 1.26 ± 0.20, 0.28 ± 0.03, and 0.35 ± 0.02 relative units/10^3 cells/day in RPMI, DMEM, and HGEM, respectively. It should be noted that the antibody titer in RPMI is somewhat higher than usual (usually 2000–3000) such that antibody productivity is normally around 0.7 relative units/10^3 cells/day. Other than this, the growth and antibody production kinetics presented here are representative.

B. Carbohydrate and Energy Metabolism

Glucose levels in RPMI and DMEM decreased markedly during exponential growth (Fig. 1, columns A and B; Table 1). Glucose utilization was accompanied by a rapid accumulation of lactate to levels (± SE) of 16.2 ± 0.8 mM and 25.3 ± 1.3 mM on cessation of growth in RPMI and DMEM media, respectively. The medium pH in RPMI declined from 7.33 to 6.84 after 69 hr and in DMEM from 7.52 to 6.87 after 97 hr, presumably due to the accumulation of lactate. In HGEM, fructose was used relatively slowly (Table 1; Fig. 1) and no net accumulation of lactate occurred (Fig. 1). Accordingly, the medium pH remained between 7.4 and 7.45 for the majority of the experiment.

In Madin Darby canine kidney cells the use of fructose instead of glucose alleviated the large decreases in pH and redox potential that normally occur as a result of lactate formation in glucose-containing medium (4). The use of fructose as an alternative carbon source to glucose stabilized pH and presumably the redox potential in HGEM cultures of anti-HT cells. However no clear improvement in antibody or growth yields was obtained.

In all three growth media glutamine was utilized more rapidly than any other amino acid (Fig. 1, Table 1). On cessation of growth, glutamine was

Table 1 Utilization and Production of Metabolites in Suspension Cultures
of anti-HT Cells

	RPMI medium			DMEM medium
	Initial conc. (mM)	% initial conc. at 69 hr[a,b]	Rate const.[c] (mmoles/cell/ hr $\times 10^{11}$)	Initial conc. (mM)
Carbohydrates				
Fructose	0.0	–	–	0.0
Glucose	10.9	15.1 (±21)	−26.7	21.5
Lactate	2.3	704.3 (±5)	+40.2	1.8
Pyruvate	0.0	(0.57) (±9)[d]	+1.6	0.79
Amino Acids				
Alanine	0.114	1538.2 (±10)	+4.7	0.130
Arginine	1.212	45.3 (±4)	−1.9	0.380
Asparigine	0.354[e]	61.0	−0.4	0.000[e]
Aspartate	0.140[e]	68.0	−0.1	0.018[e]
Cysteine	0.273	66.5 (±8)	−0.3	0.204
Glutamate	0.264	116.3 (±4)	+0.1	0.105
Glutamine	3.430	21.0 (±19)	−7.8	4.165
Glycine	0.202	68.3 (±4)	−0.2	0.448
Histidine	0.061	55.7 (ND)	−0.1	0.167
Hydroxyproline	0.143[e]	97.0	0.0	TRACE[e]
Isoleucine	0.362	35.9 (±15)	−0.7	0.729
Leucine	0.375	26.5 (±16)	−0.8	0.739
Lysine	0.220	7.3 (ND)	−0.6	0.721
Methionine	0.089	25.3 (±2)	−0.2	0.170
Phenylalanine	0.108	18.0 (±8)	−0.2	0.384
Proline	0.160	233.0 (±10)	+0.6	0.029[e]
Serine	0.267[e]	56.0	−0.3	0.389[e]
Threonine	0.175[e]	15.0	−0.4	0.789[e]

DMEM medium		Initial conc. (mM)	HGEM medium	
% Initial conc. at 97 hr[a,b]	Rate const.[c] (mmoles/cell/hr × 10^{11})		% Initial conc. at 78 hr[a,b]	Rate const.[c] (mmoles/cell/hr × 10^{11})
—	—	18.8	95.5 (±0)	−1.2
32.5 (±2)	−28.8	0.0	—	—
1419.4 (±5)	+34.6	2.1	95.6 (±2)	−0.2
34.2 (±11)	ND	0.74	16.0 (±15)	−1.3
1307.3 (±3)	+3.4	0.112	862.9 (±6)	+1.8
27.6 (ND)	−0.6	0.354	34.5 (±2)	−0.5
(0.034)[d]	+0.1	0.000[e]	(0.036)[d]	+0.1
111.1	0.0	0.018[e]	255.5	+0.1
<25.0	~0.3	0.220	34.8 (±18)	−0.3
162.4 (±1)	+0.3	0.118	308.9 (±11)	+0.5
8.3 (±1)	−7.9	4.202	3.2 (±36)	−8.6
119.0 (±0)	ND	0.401	217.2 (±3)	+1.0
57.4 (±8)	−0.1	0.129	77.5 (±1)	−0.1
TRACE	ND	TRACE[e]	TRACE	ND
34.8 (±1)	−0.9	0.788	47.6 (±2)	−0.9
27.6 (±2)	−1.0	0.779	40.6 (±4)	−1.0
57.6 (±3)	−0.6	0.718	68.9 (±1)	−0.5
38.2 (±0)	−0.2	0.188	41.5 (±12)	−0.2
64.7 (±8)	−0.6	0.368	74.0 (±3)	−0.2
972.4 (±0)	+0.4	0.029[e]	496.6	+0.2
54.7	−0.4	0.389[e]	64.0	−0.3
74.0	−0.4	0.789[e]	76.3	−0.4

Table 1   (Continued)

	RPMI medium			DMEM medium
	Initial conc. (mM)	% initial conc. at 69 hr[a,b]	Rate const.[c] (mmoles/cell/ hr $\times 10^{11}$)	Initial conc. (mM)
Amino Acids (Continued)				
Tyrosine	0.107	47.7 (±16)	−0.2	0.339
Valine	0.142	5.2 (ND)	−0.4	0.649
Ammonia	0.00	(2.97) (±1)[d]	+8.6	0.00

[a]Average values from single determinations of duplicate samples except in physiological amino acid analysis where only one sample was analyzed (see Materials and Methods). The % standard error between duplicates is shown in parenthesis. ND (not determined) designates samples where only one of the samples could be accurately determined.
[b]Cessation of growth occurred at about these times.
[c]The first order rate constant (k) for utilization (−) or production (+) of various metabolines was calculated during the growth phase in RPMI (0–69 hr), DMEM (0–73 hr), and HGEM (0–78 hr) media according to the equation of Roberts (27):

$$k = \frac{\Delta C}{T} \quad \frac{LnN - LnNo}{N - No}$$

where ΔC = change in concentrations of amino acids (mmole/L), T = time interval during which measurements were made as indicated above, No = initial cell concentration (cells/L), N = final cell concentration after time T (cells/L).
[d]Where no metabolite was present initially, the concentration (mM) of the metabolite present in culture medium on cessation of growth is shown.
[e]Since physiological amino acid analysis was not carried out on 0-hr samples of RPMI or HGEM, the starting concentrations of these amino acids were estimated as follows. In RPMI the starting concentrations were estimated from formulation data assuming a 93.5% dilution due to the addition of serum. This value was calculated by averaging the ratio of observed concentration of amino acid after addition of serum (10%) to the concentration of amino acid in the medium formulation for a number of readily quantitable amino acids. In HGEM the starting concentrations of amino acids were assumed to be the same as in DMEM.

| DMEM medium | | HGEM medium | | |
% Initial conc. at 97 hr[a,b]	Rate const.[c] (mmoles/cell/ hr $\times$ 10^{11})	Initial conc. (mM)	% Initial conc. at 78 hr[a,b]	Rate const.[c] (mmoles/cell/ hr $\times$ 10^{11})
63.9 (±11)	−0.2	0.407	78.5 (±0)	−0.2
41.1 (±5)	−0.8	0.845	56.2 (±6)	−0.8
(3.09) (±19)[d]	+4.1	0.00	(2.82) (±1)[d]	+5.5

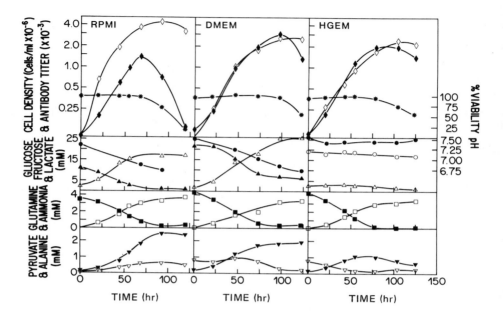

Figure 1 Growth and antibody production kinetics and nutrient levels in spinner flask cultures of anti-HT hybridoma cells in RPMI, DMEM, and HGEM are presented in columns respectively. Viable cell density (♦), antibody titer (◇), viability (*), pH (●), concentrations in the growth medium of glucose (▲), lactate (△), fructose (○), glutamine (■), ammonia (□), pyruvate (▽), and alanine (▼) were measured as described in Materials and Methods. Average values from duplicate cultures are shown.

reduced from starting levels of 3–4 mM to 0.72 ± 0.14 mM, 0.34 ± 0.00 mM, and 0.13 ± 0.05 mM in culture supernatants of RPMI, DMEM, and HGEM media, respectively. Furthermore the glutamine concentration in RPMI was reduced to 0.28 ± 0.08 mM (8%) 24 hr after cessation of growth (Fig. 1). The spontaneous degradation of glutamine (14) was estimated in spinner flasks containing DMEM in the absence of cells. Approximately 75% of starting levels of glutamine remained after 97 hr at 37°C (half-life approximately 10 days). Thus the vast majority of glutamine utilized is directly metabolized by the cells. High concentrations of ammonium accumulated in all three media (Fig. 1; Table 1). Ammonium production paralleled glutamine utilization, albeit in a nonstoichiometric manner (Table 1). If we assume that ammonium was formed from glutamine catabolism the yields were 87%, 74%, and 67% in RPMI, DMEM, and HGEM, respectively.

On replacement of glucose by fructose or galactose in cultures of HeLa cells, close to 100% of the cellular energy requirement was satisfied by glutamine catabolism (15). Even in the presence of 10 mM glucose more than half of the cell energy requirement is satisfied by glutamine. In HeLa cells the utilization rate of glutamine from medium containing 10 mM glucose was 36% as fast as from medium containing fructose or galactose. On the other hand, the utilization rates from anti-HT cultures in RPMI and DMEM are 91% and 92% as fast as from HGEM cultures (Fig. 1), which indicates that in anti-HT cells the majority of energy requirement is satisfied by glutamine even in the presence of high glucose concentrations.

Pyruvate concentrations in the medium increased in RPMI from zero to about 0.6 mM on cessation of growth (Fig. 1; Table 1). In DMEM, after a period of no net utilization, pyruvate levels dropped from about 0.8 to 0.3 mM. In HGEM, where no pyruvate was apparently formed through glycolysis, net utilization of exogenous pyruvate occurred from the outset of the experiment and dropped from 0.7 to 0.1 mM. Relatively high concentrations of alanine accumulated in all three media (Fig. 1; Table 1).

Although glucose is used three to four times faster than glutamine (Table 1), the majority of glucose is converted to lactate (some lactate may also be formed from citric acid intermediates derived primarily from glutamine) (15,16). In recent years it has become apparent that glutamine is a major energy source in several tissues and cell lines and the major product from glutamine catabolism is CO_2 (15,17–20). Consistent with these findings was that glutamine was utilized rapidly and almost completely in the cultures of anti-HT cells. The observed catabolism of glutamine and subsequent production of ammonium and alanine from HT cells suggest the following pathway:

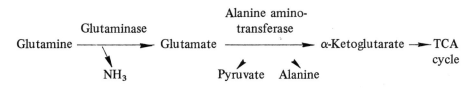

Furthermore, alanine is seen to accumulate more slowly and to a lesser extent in HGEM than in RPMI or DMEM. This may reflect the fact that since no endogenous pyruvate is being formed by glycolysis in HGEM, as evidenced by previous data (Fig. 1; Table 1), pyruvate limitation inhibits transamination between glutamate and pyruvate (21) thus limiting alanine formation. This is borne out further by the higher accumulation of glutamate in HGEM than in the other media (Table 1).

These data suggest, but do not prove, that the catabolism of glutamine results in the formation of ammonium and alanine. Absolute proof of this must await radiolabeling experiments. In fact, a major objection to this interpretation is that the rate of ammonium and alanine production is significantly less than glutamine utilization (approximately 50%). This suggests that alternative pathways of glutamine utilization may be functioning (22). Pools of glutamate can be diverted to metabolic pathways other than through alanine amino transferase. Glutamine can be metabolized by a number of known mammalian 5-aminotransferase enzymes other than glutaminase without coordinate generation of ammonium (22).

C. Amino Acid Metabolism

Table 1 shows amino acid metabolism data for anti-HT cells in RPMI, DMEM, and HGEM. Since there is a great variation among the three experiments in the exact time when cell proliferation ceases and in the original composition of amino acids, the rate of utilization and production of amino acids is employed as the primary method of comparison. In RPMI, the amino acids used most rapidly in descending order of rates of utilization were glutamine $\gg$ arginine $>$ leucine $>$ isoleucine $>$ lysine $>$ valine $>$ threonine. DMEM and HGEM are, in general, richer in amino acids than RPMI; however, the same general trends for amino acid utilization by anti-HT cells occurred in these media, with the exception of valine, which was used more rapidly, and arginine, which was used more slowly than in RPMI (Table 1).

The high utilization rates of the branched chain amino acids leucine, isoleucine, and valine along with the basic amino acids arginine and lysine, in addition to glutamine, in all media tested, suggests that these amino acids are important for the growth and antibody production of anti-HT cells. These observations are generally in good agreement with those of others working with different cell lines (23,24). In particular a nutritional study of a mouse myeloma cell line grown in Leibovitz medium (in which galactose replaces glucose) showed the same trends (25). The small number of studies carried out on amino acid utilization in tissue culture seem to indicate that there is a universal requirement for these amino acids.

The concentrations of proline, glutamic acid, and alanine increased in all three media in the course of the experiment (Table 1). In RPMI and DMEM net production of these amino acids followed the general pattern alanine $\gg$ proline $>$ glutamate. Also, glycine increased in DMEM and HGEM but not in RPMI. In HGEM glycine and glutamate accumulated to higher levels and alanine accumulated more slowly and to a lesser extent than the other media (Table 1). In RPMI no net use of hydroxyproline occurred and cysteine utilization was unusual in that it was used after 44 hr; prior to that time no net utilization was apparent.

Table 2 Growth and Antibody Yields from Individual Amino Acids

Amino acid	Growth yield[a] (cells produced/pmole of amino acid utilized)			Antibody yield[a] (antibody titer/nmole of amino acid utilized)		
	RPMI	DMEM	HGEM	RPMI	DMEM	HGEM
Arginine	1.94	6.28	7.24	5.6 (5.4)[b]	6.2	7.1
Cysteine	14.08	11.21	12.08	40.3 (19.0)	11.8	10.7
Glutamine	0.48	0.28	0.43	1.4 (1.0)	0.5	0.4
Histidine	47.70	28.12	59.76	136.6 (55.5)	27.8	56.6
Isoleucine	5.55	4.07	4.02	15.9 (9.8)	4.0	4.0
Leucine	4.68	3.63	3.76	13.4 (7.7)	3.6	3.6
Lysine	6.31	5.76	7.75	18.1 (15.1)	5.7	7.3
Methionine	19.37	19.49	15.75	55.4 (46.9)	19.3	14.9
Phenylalanine	14.55	14.29	18.15	41.7 (25.7)	14.1	17.2
Tyrosine	23.00	17.77	19.81	65.8 (48.0)	17.6	18.7
Valine	9.57	4.97	4.68	27.4 (24.1)	4.9	4.4

[a]Specific cellular and antibody yields were calculated between the time intervals 0–69 hr, 73 hr, and 78 hr in RPMI, DMEM, and HGEM, respectively. Yields were calculated by dividing the change in cell number or antibody titer over the above time intervals by the change in concentration of the respective amino acid (duplicates).
[b]Data from a different experiment in which the maximum antibody titer was 2110 (3) as opposed to 4370.

Upon cessation of growth after 69 hr in RPMI, four amino acids had been reduced to 20% or less of their initial concentrations (see Table 1; valine > lysine > threonine > phenylalanine). Of these only valine and lysine were almost completely utilized from the growth medium. Although the same general trends of amino acid utilization pertained in DMEM and HGEM, these media are rich in amino acids; thus only glutamine was reduced to significant levels on cessation of growth in both media (8% and 3%, respectively).

Table 2 shows growth and antibody yields relative to the amount of each amino acid utilized. In general, the growth yields in RPMI 1640 are equal to or slightly better than in DMEM and HGEM. However, the antibody yields in RPMI are clearly higher than in DMEM and HGEM. The maximum titer of antibody produced in RMPI in this experiment was 4370. This is higher

Table 3   Effect of exogenous Ammonium Chloride on Cell and Antibody Production in 72-hr-old Stationary Cultures

Initial conc. NH$_4$Cl (mM)	RPMI						DMEM	
	0	4	8	12	16	24	0	4
Antibody titer (%)	100 (±8) (±11)	93 (±4)	52	54 (±0)	18 (±9)	21 (±16)	100 (±13) (±4)	114 (±0)
Viable cell density (%)	100 (±6) (±0)	76 (±5)	54 (±3)	27 (±3)	28 (±1)	6 (±4)	100 (±3) (±0)	64 (±7)
Viability (%)	100 (±0) (±0)	101 (±1)	98 (±0)	76 (±7)	81 (±5)	52 (±3)	100 (±0) (±3)	94 (±7)

Average values from duplicate cultures from two separate experiments (± % standard error between duplicates)

than usual (usually 2000–3000). However even when specific antibody yields from a previous experiment, where the maximum antibody titer was 2110 (3), are considered (in parentheses in Table 2), antibody yields were still significantly higher than in DMEM and HGEM.

D. Effect of Exogenous Ammonium on Cell Proliferation and Antibody Production

Of the metabolites monitored, those that accumulate and hence are potentially toxic have been shown to be lactate (in glucose-containing medium), alanine, and ammonium. In experiments with stationary cultures (T-flask cultures) exogenous alanine up to concentrations of 16 mM had no detrimental affect on growth or antibody production from anti-HT cultures in any of the media studies (data not shown). A similar experiment was not carried out with lactate, however, since, as reported elsewhere (26), lactic acid concentrations of about 33 mM added to hybridomas at the outset of culture did not significantly affect growth or antibody production. The effect of exogenous

DMEM				HGEM					
8	12	16	24	0	4	8	12	16	24
26 (±7)	22 (±40)	9 (±0)	4 (±0)	100 (±11) (±6)	60 (±9)	10 (±0)	21 (±30)	6 (±0)	5 (±6)
37 (±7)	8 (±9)	2 (±7)	1 (±5)	100 (±1) (±2)	27 (±6)	1 (±1)	<1	<1	<1
94 (±1)	60 (±9)	29 (±0)	21 (±5)	100 (±2) (±2)	44 (±3)	19 (±33)	0 (±0)	0 (±1)	0 (±0)

ammonium chloride (NH_4Cl) on stationary cultures of anti-HT cells is shown in Table 3. RPMI and DMEM cultures in the presence of 4 mM exogenous NH_4Cl showed little or no inhibition of antibody productivity but did show some inhibition of growth. This differential affect of 4 mM ammonium chloride on proliferation and antibody production was also seen in HGEM cultures. At concentrations of NH_4Cl above 4 mM the uncoupling of antibody production from growth was not apparent and significant inhibition of both growth and antibody production was seen in all cultures. Cultures grown in HGEM clearly showed lower tolerance to exogenous NH_4Cl than those grown in RPMI and DMEM.

The levels of ammonium generated in HT cultures are less than 4 mM, so ammonium may not exert any toxic effect in these experiments. However if, as suggested above, ammonium is generated due to glutamine utilization, supplementation of batch cultures with glutamine may cause generation of toxic levels of ammonium (see a review by Dean et al. [27] for some effects of exogenous amines on mammalian cells).

IV. SUMMARY AND CONCLUSIONS

In conclusion, we have evaluated three different commercially available media for their abilities to support growth and monoclonal antibody production. The levels of antibody produced in RPMI in these experiments are unusually high (usually titers of 2000–3000/3 day culture are obtained). Normally titers comparable to those in DMEM and HGEM are obtained. Accordingly, from a production standpoint (an essential criterion for a production medium being to allow production of the highest possible level of antibody per unit time per unit volume of medium), all three media are equivalent. However, the specific productivity of antibody (antibody titer/10^3 cells/day) in a normal RPMI culture is 2–2.5 times higher than in DMEM or HGEM. This may be due to a more efficient utilization of amino acids specifically for antibody production, as reflected in higher antibody yields but equivalent growth yields in RPMI cultures compared to the other media (Table 2). Based on these data, RPMI may be the best basal medium of the three for further development of culture processes for anti-HT cells. On cessation of growth in RPMI the amino acids valine and lysine are nearly exhausted and glucose is reduced to 15% of starting levels; also, glutamine is reduced to below 10% of starting levels 24 hr after cessation of growth. Using this information it should be possible to design batch-fed processes involving supplementation of the desired nutrients to prolong growth and antibody production or antibody production in the absence of growth (28,29).

ACKNOWLEDGMENTS

We thank Marybeth Erker and Debbie Kulman for typing the manuscript, Dr. T. Pearson for a gift of the anti-HT-hybridoma cells, Alan Jones and Teresa Razniewska for developing the ammonia assay, Don Burke for performing the conventional amino acid analysis, and Floyd Snyder for the physiological amino acid analysis.

REFERENCES

1. Kohler, G. and Milstein, C. (1974). Continuous cultures of fused cells secreting antibody of predefined specificity. *Nature* (*London*) *256*: 495–497.
2. Edwards, P. A. W. (1981). Some properties and applications of monoclonal antibodies. *Biochem. J. 200*: 1–10.
3. Adamson, S. R., Fitzpatrick, S. L., Behie, L. A., Gaucher, G. M., and Lesser, B. H. (1983). In vitro production of high titre monoclonal antibody by hybridoma cells in dialysis culture. *Biotech. Lett. 5*: 573–578.

4. Imamura, T., Crespi, C. L., Thilly, W. G., and Brunegraber, H. (1982).
    Fructose as a carbon source yields stable pH and redox parameters in
    microcarrier cell culture. *Anal. Biochem. 124*: 353–358.
5. Shulman, M., Wilde, C. D., and Kohler, G. (1978). A better line for making
    hybridomas secreting antibodies. *Nature (London) 276*: 269–271.
6. Weatherburn, M. W. (1967). Phenol-hypochlorite reaction for determina-
    tion of ammonia. *Anal. Chem. 39*: 971–974.
7. Kun, E. and Kearney, E. B. (1974). Ammonia. In *Methods of Enzymatic
    Analysis*, Vol. 3. Edited by H. U. Bergmeyer. New York, Academic Press,
    pp. 1802–1806.
8. Czok, R. and Lamprecht, W. (1974). Pyruvate, phosphoenolypyruvate
    and D-glycerate-2-phosphate. In *Methods of Enzymatic Analysis*, Vol. 3.
    Edited by H. U. Bergmeyer. New York, Academic Press, pp. 1446–1451.
9. Bernet, E. and Bergmeyer, H. U. (1974). D-fructose. In *Methods in
    Enzymatic Analysis*, Vol. 3. Edited by H. U. Bergmeyer. New York,
    Academic Press, pp. 1304–1307.
10. Lund, P. (1974). Determination (of glutamine) with glutaminase and
    glutamate dehydrogenase. In *Methods in Enzymatic Analysis*, Vol. 3.
    Edited by H. U. Bergmeyer. New York, Academic Press, pp. 1719–1722.
11. Spackman, D. H., Stein, W. H., and Moore, S. (1958). Automatic recording
    apparatus for use in the chromatography of amino acids. *Anal. Chem.
    30*: 1190–1206.
12. Mondino, A., Bongiovanni, G., Fumero, S., and Rossi, L. (1972). An im-
    proved method of plasma deproteination with sulphosalicylic acid for
    determining amino acids and related compounds. *J. Chromatogr. 74*:
    255–263.
13. Seaver, S. S., Rudolph, J. L., and Gabriels, J. E. Jr. (1984). A rapid HPLC
    technique for monitoring amino acid utilization in cell culture. *Biotech-
    niques 2*: 245–260.
14. Tritsch, G. L. and Moore, G. E. (1962). Spontaneous decomposition of
    glutamine in cell culture media. *Exp. Cell. Res. 28*: 360–364.
15. Reitzer, L. J., Wice, B. M., and Kennel, D. (1979). Evidence that gluta-
    mine, not sugar, is the major energy source for cultured HeLa cells. *J.
    Biol. Chem. 254*: 2669–2676.
16. Zielke, H. R., Sumbilla, C. M., Sevdalian, D. A., Hawkins, R. L., and
    Ozand, P. T. (1980). Lactate: A major product of glutamine-metabolism
    by human diploid fibroblasts. *J. Cell Physiol. 104*: 433–441.
17. Windmueller, H. G. and Spaeth, A. E. (1974). Uptake and metabolism of
    plasma glutamine by the small intestine. *J. Biol. Chem. 249*: 5070–5079.
18. Lavietes, B. B., Regan, D. D., and Demopoulas, H. B. (1974). Glutamate
    oxidation in 6C3HED lymphoma: Effects of L-asparaginase on sensitive
    and resistant lines. *Proc. Natl. Acad. Sci. USA 71*: 3993–3997.
19. Kovacevic, A. and Morris, H. P. (1972). The role of glutamine in the oxi-
    dative metabolism of malignant cells. *Cancer Res. 32*: 326–333.

20. Donnelly, M. and Scheffler, I. E. (1976). Energy metabolism in respiration-deficient and wild type chinese hamster fibroblasts in culture. *J. Cell. Physiol. 89*: 39–52.

21. McKeehan, W. L. and McKeehan, K. A. (1983). Alanine amino transferase activity with unusually low glutamate and high pyruvate and alanine requirement in the cytosol of human fibroblasts. *In Vitro 19*: 255.

22. McKeehan, W. L. (1982). Glycolysis, glutaminolysis and cell proliferation. *Cell Biol. Int. Rep. 6*: 635–650.

23. Lambert, K. and Pirt, S. J. (1975). The quantitative requirements of human diploid cells (strain MRC-5) for amino acids vitamins and serum. *J. Cell Sci. 17*: 397–411.

24. Butler, M. and Thilly, W. G. (1982). MDCK microcarrier cultures: Seeding density effects and amino acid utilization. *In vitro 18*: 213–219.

25. Roberts, R. S., Hsu, H. W., Lin, K. D., and Yang, T. J. (1976). Amino acid metabolism of myeloma cells in culture. *J. Cell Sci. 21*: 609–615.

26. Seaver, S., Rudolph, J. L., Ducibella, T., and Gabriels, J. E. (1984). Hybridoma cell metabolism/antibody secretion in culture. In *Biotech 84*. Middlesex, U.K., Online Publication, pp. 325–344.

27. Dean, R. J., Jessup, W., and Roberts, C. R. (1984). Effects of exogenous amines on mammalian cells, with particular reference to membrane flow. *Biochem. J. 217*: 27–40.

28. Birch, J. R., Thompson, P. W., Lambert, K., and Boraston, R. (1984). The large scale cultivation of hybridoma cells producing monoclonal antibodies. Presented at the American Chemical Society, Philadelphia, 1984.

29. Flickinger, M. C., Lebherz, W. B. III, Lee, S. M., Pickle, D. J., and Hopkins, R. III. (1985). Process technologies for anticancer biologics. Presented at the Society of Industrial Microbiology, Boston, 1985.

3

Reducing Costs Upfront: Two Methods for Adapting Hybridoma Cells to an Inexpensive, Chemically Defined Serum-Free Medium

BRUCE L. BROWN
Hazleton Biotechnologies Company, Vienna, Virginia

I. INTRODUCTION

The production of monoclonal antibodies through tissue culture (1) has provided a new generation of immunologic reagents for basic research, diagnostics, and therapeutics. Depending upon its applications, the requirements for each antibody can vary from a few milligrams to kilograms.

Traditionally, hybridoma cell lines are grown in various media or combinations of media containing 5–20% fetal bovine serum (FBS) and other supplements. The ecnomics of scale-up, as well as problems and cost of purifying monoclonal antibodies from a heterologous protein backround, have necessitated the development of serum-free medium. Other problems with serum are fluctuating supply, lot-to-lot variations that can affect cellular functions, and the risk of contamination by mycoplasma, viruses, bacteria, and bacteriophage (2–8).

One of the main contaminants of FBS is bovine viral diarrhea virus (BVDV) (9). Although contamination of FBS is not a serious problem to investigators using culture systems in which the viral contaminants will not replicate, it is significant to investigators working with bovine cell culture systems. It has been shown that heat inactivation of serum at 56°C for 30 min does not eliminate BVDV from sera (9). Another aspect of using serum-free media is the cost factor. Medium containing serum costs about twice as much as medium without serum even when the serum is replaced with supplements such as insulin, transferrin, selenium, and lipoproteins.

The first part of this chapter describes an inexpensive chemically defined medium that supports the growth and maintenance of a mouse myeloma cell line suitable for use as a fusion partner. Newly formed hybrids constructed with this line will grow well in the absence of serum. Culture supernatants, even from the original fusion wells, can be screened for specific antibody production without a serum background. This is of particular importance if the target antigen is a normal component of serum.

The second part describes an on-line method for adapting a monoclonal antibody-producing cell line growing in a serum-containing medium to serum-free medium with little or no loss of antibody secretion.

II. ADAPTATION OF A MURINE MYELOMA CELL LINE TO A SERUM–FREE MEDIUM

A. Materials and Methods

1. Cell Lines and Culture Media

The myeloma cell line chosen for adaption to serum-free media for serum-free fusions was the mouse myeloma cell line P3-X63-Ag8.653 that was isolated by Kearney et al. (10) and does not express immunoglobulin heavy or light chains. This cell line is a clone from the original P3-X63-Ag8.

Iscove's Modified Dulbecco's Medium (IMDM) (Hazleton Resource Products, Denver, PA) was used throughout these studies. Its formulation is shown in Table 1. The supplements added to the media are shown in the blocked-in area. These include L-glutamine 292 mg/L; sodium pyruvate 110 mg/L, human transferrin 5 mg/L, and penicillin–streptomycin 50 IU/ml and 50 μg/ml respectively. The myeloma cell line was initially cultured in IMDM supplemented with glutamine, sodium pyruvate, antibiotics and 10% FBS. Over a period of approximately 6 weeks, the cells were adapted to serum-free growth conditions by a serial reduction of the serum and by supplementing the medium with 5 μg/ml of human transferrin as follows:

  1. Cells routinely grown in IMDM + 10% FBS; L-glutamine; Na pyruvate and antibiotics (IMDM-complete)

Table 1   Iscove's Modified Dulbecco's Medium

	mg/L		mg/L
Inorganic salts		Amino acids	
CaCl$_2$ (anhyd)	165.00	L-Alanine	25.00
KCl	330.00	L-Asparagine-H$_2$O	28.40
KNO3	0.076	L-Arginine-HCl	84.00
MgSO$_4$ (anhyd)	97.67	L-Aspartic Acid	30.00
NaCl	4505.00	L-Cystine-2HCl	91.24
NaHCO$_3$	3024.00	L-Glutamic Acid	75.00
NaH$_2$PO$_4$-H$_2$O	125.00	L-Glutamine	584.00
Na$_2$SeO$_3$-5H$_2$O	0.0173	Glycine	30.00
		L-Histidine-HCl-H$_2$O	42.00
Vitamins		L-Isoleucine	105.00
Biotin	0.13	L-Leucine	105.00
D-Ca pantothenate	4.00	L-Lysine-HCl	146.00
Choline chloride	4.00	L-Methionine	30.00
Folic acid	4.00	L-Phenylalanine	66.00
i-Inositol	7.20	L-Proline	40.00
Nicotinamide	4.00	L-Serine	42.00
Pyridoxal HCl	4.00	L-Threonine	95.00
Riboflavin	0.40	L-Tryptophane	16.00
Thiamine HCl	4.00	L-Tyrosine (disodium salt)	104.20
Vitamin B$_{12}$	0.013	L-Valine	94.00
Other components		Supplements	
D-Glucose	4500.00	L-Glutamine	292.00
Phenol red	15.00	Sodium pyruvate	110.00
HEPES	5958.00	Human transferrin	5.00
Sodium pyruvate	110.00	Penicillin–streptomycin	50/50

2. Week 1: Serum reduced to 5% and 5 μg/ml human transferrin added; cells passed twice in this media
3. Week 2: Serum reduced to 2.5% plus transferrin; cells passed twice in this media
4. Week 3: Serum reduced to 1.25% plus transferrin; cells passed twice in this media
5. Week 4: Serum reduced to 0.5% plus transferrin; cells passed twice in this media
6. Week 5: Serum omitted and the media contains 5 μg/ml of human transferrin L-glutamine, sodium pyruvate, and antibiotics (IMDM-SF).

Throughout the adaptation process, the myeloma cells (.653-SF) were maintained in 8-azaguanine at 10^4M to preserve their sensitivity to hypoxanthine, aminopterin, thymidine (HAT). After several passages in defined medium, the cell line was cloned by limited dilution in order to isolate a clonal population with a fixed growth rate.

Two clones were selected as having a stable growth rate. These were scaled-up for frozen stocks, analyzed for chromosome alteration and tested for sensitivity to HAT, and their ability to perform as fusion partners for use in monoclonal antibody production. Chromosome analysis indicated that the cell line was not altered (Table 2). The mean chromosome number for .653 (parent) was 85 and the mean chromosome number for .653-SF was 82. The 653-SF cell line was still sensitive to HAT and 95% of the cells were killed in the presence of HAT within 4 days after exposure. At this time the cell line was tested as a fusion partner with immunized spleen cells from Balb/C mice immunized with two separate immunogens.

2. Immunizations

Five mice each were immunized at 2-week intervals with 5 μg/mouse of bovine thyroglobulin (BT) (mol. wt. 660,000) or 5 μg/mouse of human placental lactogen (HPL) (mol. wt. 20,000). Each mouse received four immunizations. The fusions were performed 3 days after the final boost.

3. Cell Fusion

Two spleens from each group of immunized mice were used as the source of splenocytes for fusion with .653-SF and subsequent growth in IMDM-SF, or for fusion with .653 and subsequent growth in IMDM supplemented with 10% FBS.

The two spleens from each group were removed, minced, pooled, and washed three times in IMDM containing 2X Pen/Strep. The spleen cells were counted and divided equally into two tubes. The parent myeloma cells or the adapted cells were added to a final ratio of 4:1 (splenocytes to myeloma

Table 2 Chromosome Analysis of Cell Lines 653 and 653-SF

653

Number of cells	1	1	1	1	1	1	1	1	1	2	2	1	1	1	2
Chromosome number	51	52	53	72	80	81	83	88	90	92	94	95	97	100	101

Mean chromosome number = 85
Median chromosome number = 90–92

Markers: Two to four large metacentrics, produced by fusion at the centromere of smaller acrocentric chromosomes. A series of small accentric fragments are present in most cells.

653-SF

Number of cells	1	1	2	2	2	2	2	2	1	1	1	1
Chromosome number	52	53	60	76	83	87	88	91	92	93	96	103

Mean chromosome number = 82
Median chromosome number = 87–88

Markers: The marker chromosomes present appear the same as for cell line 653.

cells). Concurrent polyethylene-glycol- (PEG) mediated fusions were performed and the resultant hybrids were plated into 96-well Costar plates. Serum-containing or serum-free media each containing HAT were added to corresponding cultures and plates were incubated at 37°C in 95%–5% air:CO_2 atmosphere. Plates were fed at day 5 and day 10 with their respective medium containing HAT. All wells were scored for growth of hybrid colonies on day 11.

B. Results

Table 3 shows the results of the fusions of BT, a high-molecular-weight compound, and HPL, a low-molecular-weight compound, with 653 myeloma cells grown in serum-containing and serum-free IMDM. Enzyme-linked immunosorbent assay (ELISA) were used to evaluate immunoglobulin secretion and detection of antigen response to antibody that may be secreted in the microwells. Table 3 shows that in the fusion with the high-molecular-weight compound (BT) 94% and 99% of the wells tested for antibody secretion were positive in the serum-containing and serum-free fusions respectively whereas in the low-molecular-weight compound (HPL) only 8% and 3% of the wells were positive for antibody detection in the serum-containing and serum-free fusions respectively. This difference between the high-molecular-weight antigen and the low-molecular-weight antigen reflects the observed difference in the serum titers of the prefusion test bleeds (data not published).

In the serum-free fusions the percent of wells with growth was almost double in the high-molecular-weight BT fusion compared with the low-molecular-weight HPL fusion. Also, the percentage of wells positive for antigen in the BT fusions containing serum was more than 11 times that in the HPL fusion containing serum; however, in the serum-free fusions the percentage of wells positive for antigen was 33 times more in the BT fusions.

C. Discussion

The data indicate that the .653-SF cell line performs almost as well as a fusion partner as the .653 and that hybrid cells that secrete specific antibody can be constructed and maintained in an inexpensive, defined medium (IMDM) supplemented only with 5 mg/L human transferrin.

Success in either system was influenced by the molecular weight, and other unknown intrinsic factors, of the antigens used to immunize the two groups of mice. There was direct correlation between molecular weights of the immunogens with prefusion titers of the immune sera, number of splenocytes, and fusion efficiency.

Table 3 Fusion with 653 Myeloma Cells Grown in Serum-Containing and Serum-Free IMDM with Murine Splenocytes Immunized with Bovine Thyroglobulin (BT) or Human Placental Lactogen (HPL)

Fusion	No. splenocytes	No. 653	No. wells plated	No. cells/well	No. wells w/growth	No. wells assayed for antigen	No. wells positive for antigen	% of Wells positive
BT								
With 10% FBS	3.7×10^8	8.6×10^7	660	6×10^5	507	458	431	94
Without FBS	3.7×10^8	9×10^7	720	6×10^5	667	235	233	99
HPL								
With 10% FBS	1.1×10^8	2.8×10^7	480	5.8×10^5	419	419	32	8
Without FBS	1.1×10^8	2.8×10^7	480	5.8×10^5	270	270	8	3

III. ADAPTATION OF A HYBRIDOMA CELL LINE TO A SERUM–FREE, CHEMICALLY DEFINED MEDIUM

A. Materials and Methods

1. Cell Lines, Culture Media, and Growth Module

The cell line adapted to a serum-free system was a monoclonal-antibody-producing line that resulted from the fusion between immunized murine spleen cells and a murine myeloma cell line. After several clonings the resultant cell line produced 100–400 μg/ml antibody under normal growth conditions: in T-150 flasks as stationary cultures in IMDM containing 10% FBS.

The complete serum-free chemically defined media is shown in Table 1. It is Iscove's modified Dulbecco's Medium containing the additives shown in the blocked-in area.

The culture module the cells were grown in is the Millipore Cell Culture System designed for cells that continuously secrete a product. The membrane perfusion system consists of a Millipore Membrane Cell Module, 1 L medium reservoir, silicone tubing gas exchanger, and peristaltic pump (Figs. 1 and 2). The Membrane Cell Module has medium compartments and cell compartments in alternating layers (Fig. 3). Cells are trapped in the cell compartments by low-protein-binding 0.65 μm Durapore membrane. The membrane is freely permeable to proteins such as antibody and other nutrients. The cell compartments hold 12.5 ml although each compartment is so thin that no cell is further than 400 μm from the circulating medium. Medium is constantly circulated from the reservoir through a perstaltic pump to the silicone tubing gas exchanger and Membrane Cell Module and back to the reservoir. Antibody accumulates in the 1 L reservoir with the bulk of the medium and is harvested every few days by exchanging the reservoir with a new one containing fresh medium.

Operation of the system is simple. First it is primed and washed with tissue culture medium. Cells are loaded into the cell compartments of the Membrane Cell Module. Medium is circulated through the system and Membrane Cell Module via the pump. Periodically and automatically the direction of medium flow is reversed. Secreted cellular products, such as monoclonal antibody, pass through the membrane and are harvested by changing the medium in the reservoir. Antibody, nutrient, and metabolite levels can be monitored using the sample port on the reservoir. Cells are obtained by flushing medium through the cell compartment.

The antibody-secreting cells were loaded into the cell compartments of the module on day 0 at an inoculum of 8.8×10^7 cells in 300 ml complete

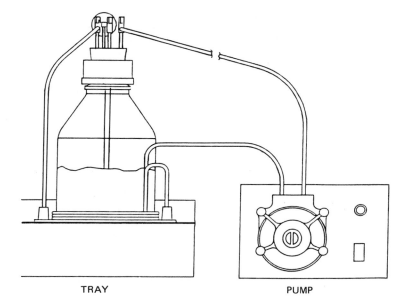

TRAY   PUMP

Figure 1   Millipore cell culture system: front view.

medium. On day 3, 700 ml of additional complete medium was added to the
reservoir and 5 days later that medium was replaced with 1000 ml of fresh
complete IMDM. This was continued on a weekly basis until day 44, at
which time the 1 L of replacement media had its serum concentration reduced
from 10% to 5% plus 5 μg/ml transferrin supplement.

At day 55 the serum concentration was further reduced to 2.5% and
supplemented with 5 μg/ml of transferrin. At day 62 the serum concentration
was further reduced to 1.25% and supplemented with 5 μg/ml transferrin. At
day 69 the serum concentration was reduced to 0% and the amount of transferrin was maintained at 5 μg/ml.

B. Results

Table 4 shows the number of days the module was on line and the amount of
antibody produced per harvest. After 204 days on line, the module lost
integrity and cells were starting to collect in the reservoir, at which point
the system was closed down.

As seen in Table 4, the amount of antibody production remained consistently high for the 103 days that the system was in the serum-free medium

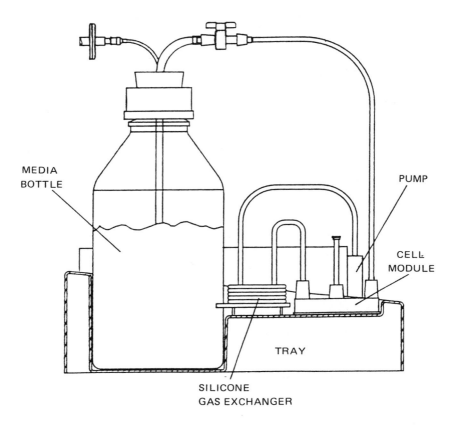

Figure 2 Millipore cell culture system: side view.

until it was closed down on the 204th day. On day 193, a sample of cells in the module was checked for viability by the trypan blue dye exclusion method. The viability was 69%. After the system was closed down, some of the cells were flushed from the module and recultured in T-75 flasks in the serum-free medium where they grew very well and were harvested and cryopreserved for another run at a later time. The total amount of antibody produced was approximately 10 g over the 204 days the system was on line as measured by radial immunodiffusion (11). The total amount of technician

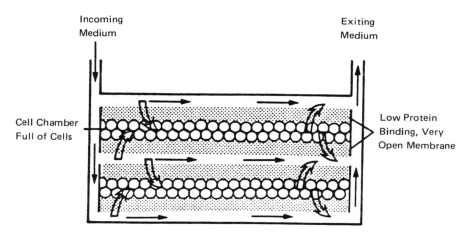

Figure 3 Internal view of the membrane-based cell perfusion system. Cells are sandwiched between two low-protein-binding microporous Durapore membranes. The narrow medium channels and open membrane promote the rapid exchange of medium between the cell compartment and medium channels. The antibody that is secreted by the cells is flushed from the cell compartment by the circulating medium.

time utilized was approximately 5.5 hr for the entire operation. The amount of antibody produced in the serum-free system was approximately 7.5 g.

C. Discussion

The adaptation of an antibody-producing cell line to a complete serum-free system is important from the point of view of purification, since it allows the purification process to be done with a minimum of steps. Also, it costs about half as much to grow cells in serum-free media such as shown here than in a serum-containing system. A third point about this system is that throughout the adaptation period the amount of antibody production did not decline and the system probably would have gone on longer if the module had not lost integrity. In addition the amount of technician time utilized throughout this complete production cycle of 204 days was approximately 5.5 hr. For the amount of product produced, this is a very good product/time ratio.

Table 4 Antibody Production in Millipore Cell Module

Days in module	Harvest no.	% Serum	Transferrin (ng/ml)	Antibody (μg/ml)
0	0	10	0	0
8	1	10	0	NA
15	2	10	0	25
22	3	10	0	104
27	4	10	0	189
31	5	10	0	231
34	6	10	0	245
38	7	10	0	293
44	8	5	5	386
50	9	5	5	386
55	10	2.5	5	340
62	11	1.25	5	416
69	12	0	5	330
76	13	0	5	318
85	14	0	5	500
89	15	0	5	350
94	16	0	5	425
100	17	0	5	425
103	18	0	5	207
109	19	0	5	318
115	20	0	5	215
122	21	0	5	451
129	22	0	5	359
135	23	0	5	414
143	24	0	5	262
150	25	0	5	373
157	26	0	5	227
165	27	0	5	480
171	28	0	5	333
178	29	0	5	507
185	30	0	5	427
193	31	0	5	375
204	32	0	5	445

IV. CONCLUSION

It has been demonstrated that there are at least two methods of reducing the costs of producing monoclonal antibodies. One was shown by adapting the parent myeloma cell line to grow in a chemically defined medium and performing the fusions with these adapted cells. The other method involved adapting a producing monoclonal antibody cell line from a serum-supplemented system to a completely serum-free system. Both of these methods are simple and straightforward.

ACKNOWLEDGMENTS

I thank Karen Shriver, Florence Nicholson, and Kathy Wheaton for their technical assistance and Donna Spiker and Pat Jenkins for help in the preparation of the manuscript.

REFERENCES

1. Köhler, G. and Milstein, C. (1975). Continuous cultures of fused cells secreting antibody of predefined specificity. *Nature 256*: 495–497.
2. Kniazeff, A. J., Wopschall, L. J., Hopps, H. E., and Morris, C. S. (1975). Detection of bovine viruses in fetal bovine serum used in cell culture. *In Vitro 11*: 400–403.
3. Molandex, C. A., Kniazeff, A. J., Boone, C. W., Paley, A., and Imagava, D. T. (1972). Isolation and characterization of viruses from fetal calf serum. *In Vitro 7*: 168–173.
4. Barile, M. F., Hopps, H. E., Grabowski, M. W., Riggs, D. B., and DelGiudice, R. A. (1973). The identification and source of mycoplasma isolated from contaminated cell cultures. *Ann. NY Acad. Sci. 225*: 251–264.
5. Orr, H. C., Sibinovic, K. H., Probst, P. G., Hochstein, H. D., and Littlejohn, D. C. (1975). Bacteriological activity in unfiltered calf serum collected for tissue culture use. *In Vitro 11*: 230–233.
6. Merril, C. R., Friedman, T. B., Attallah, A. F., Geier, M. R., Krell, K., and Yarkin, R. (1972). Isolation of bacteriophages from commercial sera. *In Vitro 8*: 91–93.
7. Moody, E. E. M., Trousdale, M., Jorgenson, G. H., and Shelokov, A. (1975). Bacteriophages and endotoxin in licensed live virus vaccines. *J. Infect. Dis. 13*: 588–591.
8. Cleveland, W. L., Wood, I., and Erlanger, B. F. (1983). Routine large-scale production of monoclonal antibodies in a protein-free culture medium. *J. Immun. Methods 56*: 221–234.
9. Rossi, C. R., Bridgman, C. R., and Kiesel, G. K. (1980). Viral contamination of bovine fetal lung cultures and bovine fetal serum. *Am. J. Vet Res. 41*: 1680–1681.

10. Kearney, J. F., Radbruch, A., Leisegang, B., and Rajewsky, K. (1979). A new mouse myeloma cell line that has lost immunoglobulin expression, but permits the construction of antibody-secreting hybrid cell lines. *J. Immunol. 123*: 1548.

11. Mancini, G., Carbonaro, A. O., and Hereman, J. F. (1965). Immuno-chemical quantitation of antigens by single radial immunodiffusion. *Immunochemistry 2*: 235.

4

Culture Method Affects Antibody Secretion of Hybridoma Cells

SALLY S. SEAVER
Hygeia Sciences, Newton, Massachusetts

I. INTRODUCTION

In the 10 years since one was first created by Kohler and Milstein (1), hybridoma clones secreting monoclonal antibodies have been made in thousands of laboratories and are being used in research, diagnostics, and therapy. As more uses are found for monoclonal antibodies, more antibody must be produced. Initially mice were the preferred method for producing "large" amounts of antibody (2). Recently, several in vitro methods, such as stirred fermentors (3–5), air-lift fermentors (6), hollow fiber cartridges (7–9), ceramic logs (10), porous beads or capsules (11), and even a large array of roller bottles have been used to produce monoclonal antibody. In the first two and last method cells are moving freely in the medium. In the other methods cells are immobilized within a matrix.

Users/manufacturers of these new systems have often claimed that the productivity of a hybridoma cell line increases in their system because large amounts of antibody (sometimes at very high concentrations) are produced. It is difficult for a user to choose a particular system based on these claims, since the amount of antibody secreted by different hybridoma lines using identical medium and culture conditions can vary almost 100-fold.

In this chapter the effect of the culture method on antibody secretion is measured using the same two hybridoma cell lines in two different small-scale

Most of the data reported in this chapter were the result of work done at Millipore Corp., Bedford, Massachusetts.

culture systems: the traditional stirred culture in a glass vessel and an experimental membrane-based perfusion system. In the first system cells are in constant motion; in the second they are immobilized between layers of membranes. Since most scale-up work begins by determining the growth, secretion, and metabolic characteristics of a cell line in static culture, these two hybridoma lines were also characterized in small dishes.

II. MATERIALS AND METHODS

A. Cell Lines and Media

The two hybridoma cell lines were fusion products of mouse spleen cells with either SP 2/0-Ag-14 myeloma (SP 2/0 hybridoma) or P3-NS1-Ag-4-1 myeloma (NS-1 hybridoma). The SP 2/0 secreted an IgG_{2a} antibody; the NS-1 hybridoma secreted an IgG_1 antibody. Both lines were routinely cultured in Dulbecco's Modified Eagle Medium containing 4.5 g/L of glucose, 10 mM Hepes at pH 7.1, 8 mM glutamine (total concentration), 100 U/ml penicillin, and 100 μg/ml streptomycin. Unless stated otherwise, 8% fetal bovine serum (Microbiological Associates or Sterile Systems) was added. The NS-1 hybridoma required 0.1 mM hypoxanthine and 16 μM thymidine.

Cell number was determined using a hemacytometer. Trypan blue was used to determine cell viability.

B. Antibody Assay

Antibody levels were determined using a full sandwich ELISA assay that was specific for mouse IgG antibody (12). Absolute concentrations of SP 2/0 antibody were determined by running affinity-purified SP 2/0 antibody as a standard on the same plate. Relative titers of NS-1 antibody were reported as the dilution titer at 50% maximum response.

C. Nutrient/Metabolite Assays

Glucose and lactic acid levels were determined by enzymatic assay (Sigma). Primary amino acid were quantified by HPLC after precolumn derivatization with ortho-phthalaldehyde (12).

D. Culture Methods

Stationary culture experiments were done in 35 mm dishes. Stirred culture experiments were performed in a Techne MSC system in a 37°C CO_2 incubator. The caps on the side arms were loosened to promote gas exchange.

In the continuous stirred culture experiment medium was changed by centrifuging the cells for 10 min at 1000 rpm in a Sorvall RC5C and resuspending them in fresh medium. Cell viability decreased less than 3% during the medium change. In this experiment a 7% CO_2/93% air mixture was continuously passed through the head space. FG Millexes (0.2 μ, Millipore Corp.) were used to filter the incoming and exiting air streams. This promoted a much faster equilibration of gas in the medium with that of the incubator.

The membrane perfusion system consisted of a membrane cell module, a silicone tubing gas exchanger, a 1 L glass medium reservoir, and a peristaltic pump that circulated the medium between the three components (see Chapter 3, Figures 1 and 2 for drawings of the system). The membrane cell module consisted of layers of membrane that divided the module into compartments through which the medium circulated and compartments in which the cells were located (Fig. 1). The membrane separating the two compartments was low-protein-binding hydrophilic Durapore (0.65 μm, Millipore Corp.). This membrane is freely permeable to all nutrients, metabolites, and particles less than 0.5 μm, including monoclonal antibody. The total volume of cell compartments was 12.5 ml. No cell was further than 400 μm from the circulating medium. The height of the medium compartment was minimized so that convection and not diffusion was the main mechanism by which medium was exchanged between the two types of compartments.

Cells (1-5 $\times$ 10^7) were seeded into the cell compartments of the membrane cell module in a fully primed system. The system was run in a CO_2 incubator. The peristaltic pump circulated medium between the three components (reservoir, gas exchanger, and cell module) at 40 ml/min. The direction of flow automatically reversed itself every 2 hr. Preliminary experiments showed that reversing the flow prolonged operation and increased antibody production. The medium was changed once or twice a week by changing the reservoirs. The antibody was harvested by changing the reservoirs since the cell compartment membranes were completely permeable to it and since the reservoir contained 94% of the medium.

The rate of antibody production in stationary or stirred culture was determined by fitting a second-order polynomial to the antibody accumulation curve. The slope of this curve divided by the number of viable cells present (which equals the rate) was determined on at least 3 different days. The rate of antibody production is expressed as the antibody produced per day per 10^6 cells. The rate of antibody production in the membrane perfusion system was determined after the number of cells in the membrane module had reached a steady state (day 14–17). The cell number was determined by removing an aliquot of the cells or by flushing the cells from the

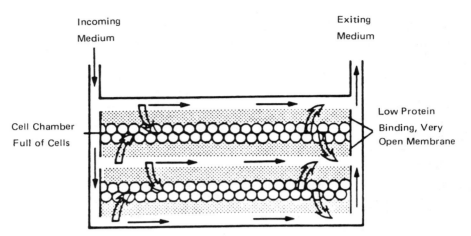

Figure 1   Internal, cross-sectional view of the membrane cell module.   Cells, represented by large circles are trapped between two layers of microporous, low-protein-binding Durapore membrane (represented by array of small dots). Medium is pumped into the membrane cell module, down the media compartments (thin arrows) and exits. Media also perfuses across the membrane into the cell compartments.

module.   The rate of antibody accumulation was determined by sampling the reservoir daily.   Results are the average of at least three different measurements.   Attempts to use the total number of cells instead of the number of viable cells to compute production rates did not yield results that could be averaged.

III.   RESULTS OF STATIONARY, STIRRED, AND PERFUSION CULTURES

A.   Stationary Culture

Stationary culture in dishes or flasks has a very limited potential for scale-up even at the pilot stage.   However, stationary culture in small dishes can be very useful for rapidly characterizing the rates of cellular proliferation, antibody secretion, consumption of nutrients, and production of metabolites as well as the optimal serum concentration for a particular cell line.   Since it is the only culture method common to all laboratories, stationary culture also has been used to compare different cell lines.   We have used stationary culture in dishes to determine the rates of cellular proliferation, antibody secretion, consumption of nutrients, and production of metabolites for both hybridoma lines.

When seeded in small dishes or flasks at 5×10^4 cells/ml, the Sp 2/0 hybridoma cells reproducibly divided rapidly ($t_D = 13 \pm 2$ hr) until cell densities reached 2-3×10^6 cells/ml (Fig. 2A). The NS-1 hybridoma cells reproducibly divided rapidly ($t_D = 15 \pm 2$ hr) when plated at 1×10^5 cells/ml and ceased dividing when cell densities were 1-2×10^6 cells/ml (Fig. 3A). The rates of proliferation are very typical for Sp 2/0- and NS-1-derived hybridomas, which normally have doubling times of 10-18 hr (our unpublished observations). The initial seeding density required for reproducible, rapid proliferation does vary among hybridoma cell lines. It usually corresponds to the initial seeding density required by the myeloma partner. Most hybridoma cell lines plateau at 1-3×10^6 cells/ml but this level can also depend on the myeloma partner used.

Antibody levels plateaued 2-3 days after cells ceased proliferating in both cases. Cell viability also remained high for 3-4 days after proliferation had ceased. The time between the end of proliferation, the start of decreased viability, and the peak in antibody levels depends on the particular hybridoma. In other hybridoma lines derived from the same myeloma cell lines, antibody levels reached their peak value within 24 hr after the cessation of cell proliferation. Cell viability can also start decreasing as soon as the cells stop proliferating. This earlier decrease occurs even when these other hybridoma lines are cultured in the same medium used here.

When this work was initiated, there were no published data on cell metbolism or even what compounds should be quantified. Since hybridoma cells are cultured in medium containing high levels of glucose, the levels of glucose and lactic acid, a common glucose metabolite, were measured. Amino acid levels were also quantified to determine if antibody production and cell proliferation were inhibited by the consumption of critical amino acids.

Hybridoma cells consumed glucose at a much faster rate during proliferation than after proliferation had stopped (Fig. 2B, C). The ratio of lactic acid production to glucose use was constant except during the initial proliferation, and averaged 1.5. If all the glucose were degraded through the Embden-Meyerhoff pathway, the ratio would be 2.0.

It has been suggested that lactic acid inhibits cell proliferation and product secretion (13). This hypothesis was based on the observation that lactic acid levels are high in mature, nonproliferating cultures. No experiments were done to show that high levels of lactic acid inhibit proliferation or secretion in freshly seeded cultures. The highest level of lactic acid measured by us for these hybridoma cell lines in any culture system was 33 mM (3 mg/ml). Therefore, we compared the effect of 33 mM lactic acid on cell proliferation

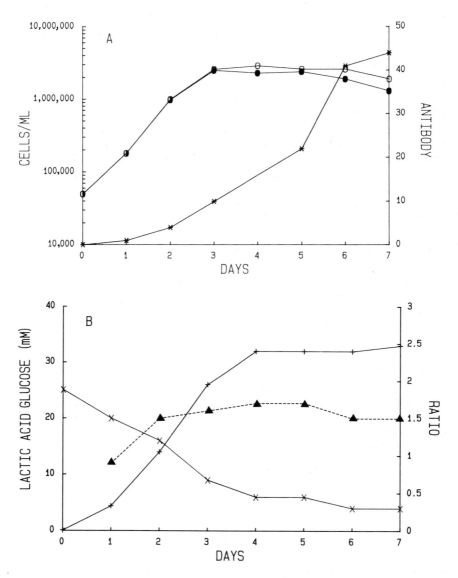

Figure 2   Sp 2/0 hybridoma line in stationary culture. A. Total cells/ml (○),
viable cells/ml (●), and antibody concentration (μg/ml, *). Antibody accumulation is plotted linearly; cell proliferation is plotted logarithmically. B. Lactic
acid (+), glucose (x), and ratio of lactic acid production to glucose use (▲).
C. Glutamine (+), alanine (x), and the ratio of glutamine to alanine (▲).

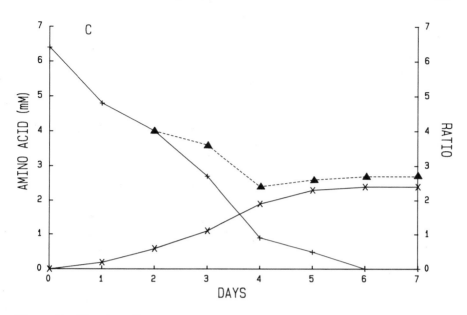

Figure 2 (Continued)

and antibody production when these hybridoma lines were seeded at low and high density. No significant effect on antibody production or the rate of cell proliferation was observed (results not shown). Similar results have been obtained by others (14). Therefore, determinations of lactic acid levels were not continued on a routine basis.

The only primary amino acids that showed dramatic changes in their levels were glutamine and alanine (Figs. 2C, 3C, 4) (12). Glutamine was rapidly consumed even after cell proliferation had ceased and until it was exhausted from the medium. Glutamine has been reported to be an alternative energy source (15). Almost all of the decrease was due to the consumption by cells and not its degradation spontaneously or by enzymes in the serum (12,16,17). The half-life of glutamine at 37°C in the medium used, Dulbecco's modified Eagle's medium with 8% fetal bovine serum, was 6.7 ± 0.5 days (12).

Alanine levels increased during culture. The production of alanine is a common phenomenon. Several other types of cells produce alanine in culture (18–20). The increase in alanine could be related to the decrease in glutamine. Glutamine can be broken down and converted to alanine via the tricarboxylic acid cycle and alanine aminotransferase (18). Since the ratio of

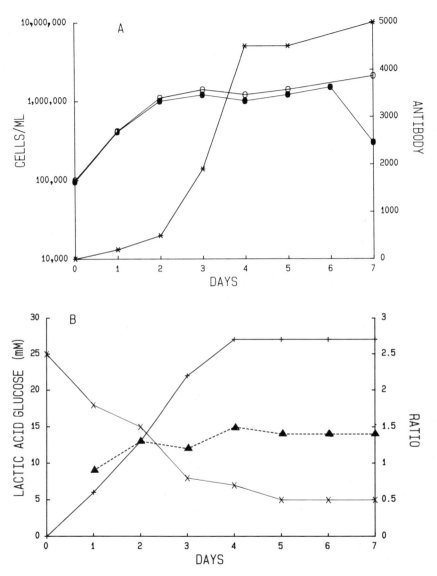

Figure 3 NS-1 hybridoma line in stationary culture. A. Total cells/ml (○),
viable cells/ml (●), and antibody concentration (arbitrary titer units, *).
Antibody accumulation is plotted linearly; cell proliferation is plotted logarithmically. B. Lactic acid (+), glucose (x), and ratio of lactic acid production to
glucose use (▲). C. Glutamine (+), alanine (x), and the ratio of glutamine to
alanine (▲).

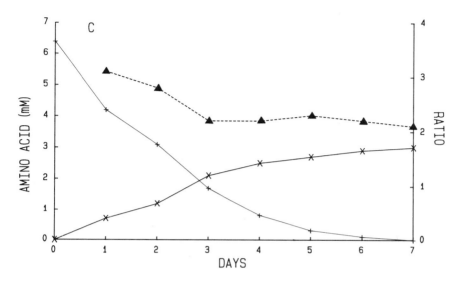

Figure 3 (Continued)

glutamine to alanine was never lower than 2.1, a maximum of 45% of the glutamine was converted into alanine by these hybridoma cells.

Glucose and glutamine are the two nutrients that in all experiments were rapidly depleted from the culture by day 4 or 5. However, adding extra glucose or glutamine on day 4 did not increase the final cell density or antibody production. There is evidence that in stirred culture adding both extra glucose and glutamine increases antibody productivity (21).

B. Traditional Stirred Culture

Two different protocols are commonly used by cell culturists when doing stirred culture. In the first cells are seeded directly into the final volume of culture fluid. In the second cells are seeded into a fraction of the final volume. Fresh medium is then added at intervals until the final volume is reached. We used both protocols with the two hybridoma cell lines. For the second protocol cells were seeded at the same density as used in the first protocol but in half the final volume. On day 3 fresh medium but no cells were added to bring the final volume to that of the first protocol. In both protocols the final volume filled only half the vessel, to allow for gas exchange. Even with the caps on the side arms loosened, this method does probably not

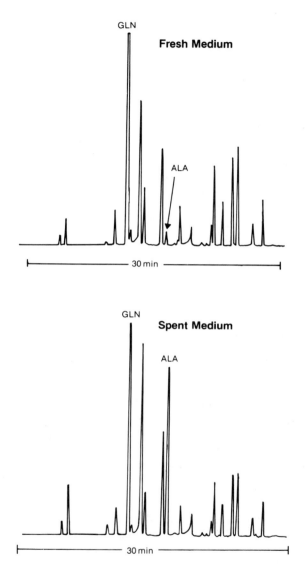

Figure 4 Profile of primary amino acids in media before and after culturing hybridoma cells. The concentration of glutamine (GLN) was 6.2 mM in the fresh medium and 1.2 mM in the spent medium. The concentration of alanine (ALA) was 0.1 mM in the fresh medium and 1.7 mM in the spent medium.

provide adequate gas exchange (see below). In both protocols the cultures were terminated after 11–12 days (total culture time).

The two hybridoma cell lines behaved very differently in stirred culture. With the Sp 2/0 hybridoma there was no difference in final cell density, viability, or antibody produced between the two protocols tried (Fig. 5). Antibody levels peaked as soon as cellular proliferation had ceased at 10–25% of the level normally reached in stationary culture. Cell viability also started to decrease as soon as proliferation ceased. The final cell density was similar to that normally found in stationary culture.

With the NS-1 hybridoma the absolute number and percentage of viable cells was higher in the second protocol: the fed-batch protocol (Fig. 6). However, the amount of antibody produced was 50% lower using this protocol. Thus, optimizing the number of viable cells does not always result in optimizing antibody production. With both protocols antibody production in stirred culture was only 50–75% of that normally found in stationary culture. As with the Sp 2/0 hybridoma, cell viability did not remain high after proliferation had finished. Unlike the Sp 2/0 hybridoma line, the NS-1 line, as has been showed with other hybridoma lines (4), continued to secrete antibody after proliferation had ceased. Other hybridoma cell lines have produced more antibody in stirred culture when the culture was converted from a batch culture to a fed-batch culture (21).

Nutrient usage/production was very similar to that measured in the stationary cultures (results not shown) (22) and by others (23). Glucose and glutamine were consumed two to four times faster during cellular proliferation than after proliferation had ceased. Alanine levels increased most rapidly during proliferation. The pattern of nutrient usage among the four stirred culture experiments was so similar that it could not account for the concomitant cessation of antibody production and cellular proliferation in the Sp 2/0 hybridoma stirred cultures (Fig. 5).

C. Perfusion Culture

Many normal eukaryotic cells have a proliferative phase and a stationary, differentiated phase in which specialized products are made. Most cells consume nutrients much faster during the proliferative than during the production phase. The main advantage of perfusion culture is to maintain the cells in the differentiated, production phase and thereby increase the amount of product secreted (per cell per unit time and per ml medium). Whether this could be routinely done with hybridoma lines was not known. Hybridoma cells are not normal eukaryotic cells; they do not have distinct proliferative and productive phases.

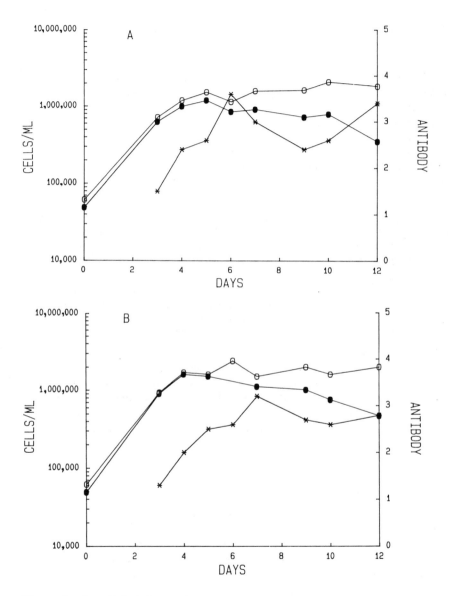

Figure 5 Sp 2/0 hybridoma line in stirred culture. A. Method A: batch culture with cells seeded into the final volume of culture medium. B. Method B: fed-batch culture with cells seeded into half the final volume of culture medium. The rest of the culture medium was added on day 3. Total cells/ml (○), viable cells/ml (●), and antibody concentrations (μg/ml, *).

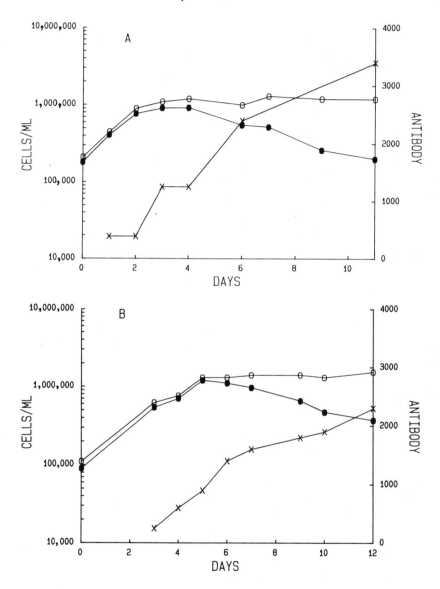

Figure 6 NS-1 hybridoma line in stirred culture. A. Method A: batch culture with cells seeded into the final volume of culture medium. B. Method B: fed-batch culture with cells seeded into half the final volume of culture medium. The rest of the culture medium was added on day 3. Total cells/ml (○), viable cells/ml (●), and antibody concentrations (arbitrary titer units, x).

In the cell module of our experimental perfusion system, cells were trapped between two membrane sheets (Fig. 1). Medium from the reservoir was pumped through a gas exchanger, through the cell module on the other side of the membrane sheets from the cells, and back to the reservoir. The cell module was very compact; the reservoir held 95% of all the medium in the system.

Superficially this perfusion system looked like a hollow fiber system with media pumped through the lumen of the fibers and cells growing on the extracapillary side of the fibers. However, there were several important differences. First, the membranes used in the perfusion system were not ultra-filtration membranes, which retain higher-molecular-weight proteins. They were microporous (0.65 μm) membranes freely permeable to all molecules including the monoclonal antibody, but retained the 15+ μm hybridoma cells. Convection and not diffusion was the main way by which molecules were exchanged between the media and the cell mass. Second, the spacing between the membrane was tightly controlled. No cell was further than 400 μm from the rapidly circulating medium. Third, the media flowed across the width of the module and not the length. Flowing across the width minimized the depletion of critical nutrients such as oxygen in the circulating medium. The cells near the side from which the media enter were not exposed to a much richer medium than the cells near the media exit port. The media flow was also periodically reversed to help maintain uniformity. Fourth, antibody was not concentrated with the cells. Antibody was harvested by changing the reservoir since 95% of the medium was in the reservoir.

The questions addressed with the perfusion system were how long the two hybridoma lines would continue to secrete antibody, what happened to cell viability and antibody production once the cells stopped proliferating, what the maximum cell densities were, and what happened when the concentration of serum was reduced. Figure 7 shows antibody production by the Sp 2/0 hybridoma in the perfusion system. Cells (1 X 10^7) were loaded in the cell module of a system primed with 300 ml medium. On day 5, 700 ml medium were added. On day 8, 1 L medium was harvested and replaced with 1 L fresh medium. Medium was replaced every 2–4 days after that.

The rate of antibody production stabilized after day 10. The amount and concentration of antibody produced depended on the rate at which the medium was replaced. It ranged from 25 to 80% of the titers normally found in the stationary culture experiment ($\sim$20 μg/ml). From this and other experiments that monitored glucose and glutamine levels, it was determined that most hybridoma lines would continue to produce as long as the level of glucose was maintained above 11 mM (1 mg/ml) and the level of glutamine above 1 mM. For the Sp 2/0 cell line, that meant changing the medium every

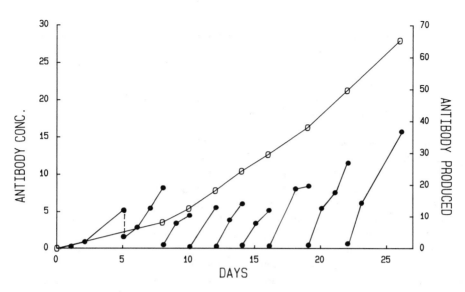

Figure 7 Sp 2/0 hybridoma antibody production in the perfusion system. Total accumulated antibody (mg, ○) and antibody concentration (μg/ml, ●). The break in the antibody concentration indicates when the antibody in the medium was harvested and fresh medium was added. The dashed line at day 5 indicates when an additional 700 ml medium was added to the original 300 ml in the system.

3–4 days, thereby harvesting 10–15 mg antibody. The Sp 2/0 hybridoma continued to secrete antibody until day 49 when the experiment was terminated. In other experiments cells secreted antibody for at least 3 months. Similar results were obtained with the NS-1 hybridoma line (see Fig. 8) and other cell lines (24).

From this and other experiments it was determined that most of the cellular proliferation occurred during the first 10–17 days. By day 14 there were 3×10^9 cells in the module at a concentration of 2.4×10^8/ml. Their viability depended on the hybridoma line (see below). This experiment also tested the effects of lowering serum concentration on the perfusion culture. The Sp 2/0 hybridoma was initially seeded in medium containing 8% fetal bovine serum, the medium in which it was routinely passaged in stationary culture. By day 8 the serum concentration in the medium had been reduced to 3% and on day 14 it was reduced to 2%. This fourfold reduction in serum had no affect on the rate of antibody production (Fig. 7).

After 3-4 weeks the viability of the cells was often low. The exact viability depended on the cell line (24) (our unpublished observations) and ranged between 30 and 90%. Therefore, the feasibility of periodically flushing the cells from the cell module and thereby maintaining high cell viability was examined. Even after a thorough flushing, approximately 5×10^7 cells remain in the module attached to the membrane. These cells quickly repopulate the cell module.

A cell module was seeded with 3×10^7 NS-1 hybridoma cells that were 82% viable. On day 16, 2×10^9 cells that were 30% viable were flushed from the cell module. Fresh medium was added to the reservoir. The rate of antibody production after flushing the cells from the module was compared to the production during the 4 days prior to the cell flushing (Fig. 8). After flushing the cell module, it took 10 days for the antibody titer to reach the levels obtained in the 4 days before the module was flushed. Similar results were obtained in repeat experiments and with other hybridoma cell lines. Even though cells had a lower viability before the flushing, there were so many more viable cells producing antibody that more antibody could be made in a shorter amount of time. After flushing, the viability was higher but there were fewer cells present so the amount of antibody produced was lower. Most of the nutrients in the medium were being used for cell proliferation and not antibody production. Therefore, periodically flushing cells from the module to maintain a high viability lowers the total amount of antibody produced in a given time period.

A second reason for wanting to maintain high cell viability is to minimize antibody degradation. Even in the cases where viability was below 50%, the antibody produced was functionally no different from that produced in cultures that maintained high viability. This is not surprising. Functional antibody has been produced routinely from stirred cultures that were not stopped until cell viability was well below 50%.

D. Direct Comparison of Stirred and Perfusion Cultures

Although the rate of antibody production per cell can be calculated for the same cell lines in stirred and perfusion culture (see below), it is difficult to compare the two methods because the conditions were not identical. The stirred cultures were batch processes while the perfusion cultures were maintained for long periods of time by periodically replacing the medium. The perfusion culture system included a gas exchanger so that the circulating medium was continuously equilibrated with the incubator. The stirred culture system had no special provision to facilitate gas exchange; the vessels were only half full so that gases in the media could exchange with those in the head space.

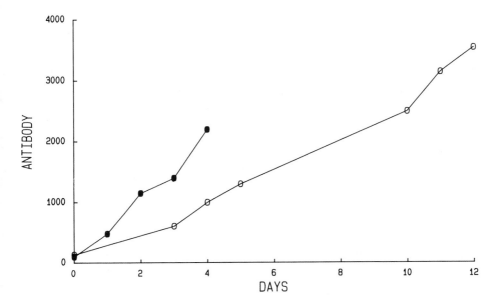

Figure 8   Effects of flushing NS-1 hybridoma cells from the cell module on antibody production. Antibody production before the cells were flushed from the module (arbitrary titer units, ●) and after cells were flushed from the module (arbitrary titer units, ○).

For a more direct comparison of the two culture methods, the stirred culture was converted to a continuous culture. Both systems were seeded with the same number of Sp 2/0 hybridoma cells in the same (total system) volume. Medium was changed at the same day. In the perfusion system medium was changed by exchanging a reservoir of spent medium with a reservoir full of fresh medium. In the stirred culture cells were gently centrifuged and resuspended in fresh medium. The centrifugation was optimized so that cell viability decreased less than 3%. Finally, gas exchange in the stirred culture vessels was also improved by flowing a mixture of 95% air and 5% CO_2 through the headspace.

Cellular proliferation lasted about 12 days in both systems, during which time similar amounts of antibody were produced (Fig. 9). After proliferation ceased, the antibody concentration in the harvested medium remained constant but at different levels for the two methods. The average concentration of antibody was 5.8 ± 1 $\mu g/ml$ in the stirred culture and 11 ± 0.4 $\mu g/ml$ in the perfusion system. This twofold difference resulted in 40 mg antibody being produced in the perfusion system by day 23 while only 23 mg was

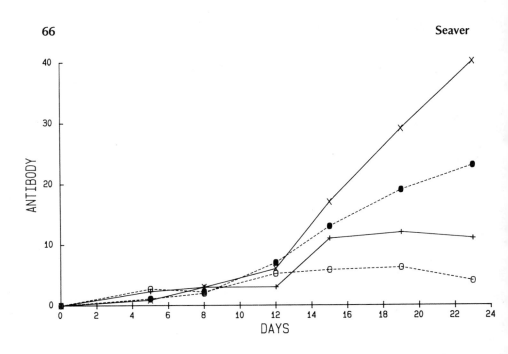

Figure 9   Side-by-side comparison of stirred and perfusion culture using the Sp 2/0 hybridoma line. Perfusion culture: total accumulated antibody (mg, x), antibody concentration (μg/ml, +). Stirred culture: total accumulated antibody (mg, ●), antibody concentration (μg/ml, ○).

made in continuous stirred culture. The Sp 2/0 hybridoma was more productive in perfusion culture.

E. Comparison of the Rates of Antibody Production

Clearly the two hybridoma cell lines behaved differently in the different culture systems. One way to quantify these differences is to compare the systems in side-by-side experiments. As the experiment described above, such side-by-side comparisons often involve major modifications of one of the culture methods. Another way to compare the efficiency of a given hybridoma line in different culture systems is to determine the rate of antibody production per cell per unit time. Table 1 shows the rate of antibody production for both cell lines in stationary, stirred, and perfusion culture. No production rate could be calculated for the Sp 2/0 hybridoma in the traditional stirred culture. Antibody production ceased early in the experiment, as soon as cellular proliferation ceased. When gas exchange was improved and the

Table 1   Rate of Antibody Production[a]

Culture system	Sp 2/0 hybridoma (μg Ab/10^6 cells/day)	NS-1 hybridoma (Ab titer/10^6 cells/day)
Stationary	4.1 ± 1.0	1000 ± 200
Stirred		
Method A[b]	n.d.[c]	490 ± 75
Method B	n.d.	243 ± 8
Continuous[d]	2.4 ± 0.3	—
Perfusion		
Batch change	6.6 ± 1.7	1300 ± 400
Continuous[d]	7.4 ± 1.0	—

[a]All calculations are in terms of viable cell number.
[b]Method A, cells were seeded in final volume; method B, cells were seeded in half the final volume: extra medium was added on day 3.
[c]Not calculated because cells ceased producing antibody as soon as they ceased proliferating.
[d]From side-by-side comparison of the stirred culture with the perfusion system.

medium was changed periodically, the Sp 2/0 hybridoma cells continued to secrete antibody after cellular proliferation stopped. Even so, the rate of antibody production in stirred culture was only 33% of that in perfusion culture and 60% of that in stationary culture. The rate of antibody production was 160% higher in perfusion culture than in stationary culture.

For the NS-1 hybridoma the rate of antibody production was similar in perfusion and stationary culture. It was 50–75% lower in stirred culture. The rate of antibody production for the two different ways of running stirred culture differed by a factor of 2. The total amount of antibody produced by batch stirred culture (method A) was 1.5 times that produced in the fed-batch cultures (method B). The total amount of antibody produced equals the rate of antibody production (per cell per day) times the total number of viable cell-days. On the average the number of viable cells was 133% higher in method B than in method A.

These data highlight two other points. First, despite the impossibility of scaling-up stationary culture, the rate of antibody production in stationary culture can be as good as or better than the rate of production in other scalable methods of culture. A two- to fourfold increase in antibody production rate is needed to make the stirred culture system as productive as the stationary or perfusion systems. Second, the data from the NS-1 hybridoma in traditional stirred culture illustrate the danger of using only the total number of viable cells to optimize antibody production methods. The total amount of antibody produced is the product of the rate of antibody production and the number of viable cell-days.

IV. DISCUSSION

We have shown that the culture method can affect the productivity of hybridoma cells, whether productivity is measured in terms of the quantity of antibody produced per cell per unit time (Table 1) or the quantity of antibody produced per ml medium used. Furthermore, the culture method affects the two hybridoma cell lines differently.

We have also found that the most important parameter to measure when optimizing antibody production is antibody production. Other substances such as nutrient consumption, metabolite production, or total viable cells may parallel antibody production but they do not predict it. This was most dramatically shown in the stirred culture experiment where the fed-batch method of propagation (method B) resulted in 33% more viable cells than batch propagation (method A) but 50% less antibody. We had previously found that the ratio of the rate of antibody production to the rate of nutrient usage or metabolite production increased when cellular proliferation ceased (22).

These other parameters are important to monitor because they can explain why certain optimization protocols work and can help establish reproducible conditions for culture. The depletion of glutamine is a reasonable explanation for the cessation of antibody production (Figs. 2 and 3). The addition of glutamine alone may not prolong antibody production. Other nutrients may also be limiting. Monitoring glutamine or glucose levels in the perfusion culture helped us establish a schedule for media changes that maintained the culture for extended periods of time.

The two different hybridoma cell lines adapted readily to a perfusion culture in which they were trapped between two layers of microporous membrane. They continued to produce antibody for weeks after they reached their maximum cell density. Similar results have been obtained with other hybridomas (24). The only way to stop the hybridoma cells from secreting antibody is to stop feeding the cells, either by stopping the circulation of the medium or by not changing the medium frequently enough. Medium was changed periodically to maintain the levels of glutamine above 1 mM and/or glucose above 11 mM (1 mg/ml). Maintaining these levels helped the culture medium from becoming seriously depleted in any critical nutrients. Antibody productivity may be increased further by continuous feeding of new medium as antibody-laden medium is withdrawn. Continuous feeding/bleeding usually increases productivity (10,21).

Hybridoma cells adapt well to a variety of perfusion systems. These include trapping the cells in alginate (25), microcapsules (11), extracapillary space of hollow fibers (7-9), pores of ceramic cartridges (10), and even in stirred cultures equipped with spin filters to remove the medium (21). In every case cells continue to secrete antibody for weeks after most proliferation has ceased. Perfusion culture allows one to "force" hybridoma cells in a nonproliferating production stage. One major benefit of perfusion cultures is the increase in productivity (10,21). A second is that after an initial phase of cellular proliferation the serum requirement of the cells is lowered dramatically (10,21,24; Fig. 7). Both these benefits help to lower production costs and simplify purification.

The best way to choose a method for scaling-up monoclonal antibody production is to compare the productivity of the particular hybridoma line in the different systems. Since it is never possible to try all the different systems, it is always tempting to try those systems for which the most fantastic claims of productivity (in terms of g antibody/day) are given. These claims are misleading because they do not state antibody productivity in normalized terms, such as amount of antibody/cell/unit time or amount of antibody/unit cost. A system that has 10^{10} cells should produce 10,000 times more antibody than a 1 ml culture (where production is expressed as $\mu g/ml$) or 10 times more than a 1 L culture. The real question is whether the fantastic system requires 30 times more medium or twice as much labor as the 1 L culture.

Such claims are also meaningless if they do not refer to the productivity of the same hybridoma in some standard system or the productivity of some standard cell line in the fantastic system. To date there is no standard hybridoma line. Several "standard" systems are available to any culture laboratory. The most common is stationary culture in small dishes or flasks, followed by culture in roller bottles or stirred culture. However, such comparisons can be difficult. The amount of antibody secreted/cell/unit time by either hybridoma studied was two to four times higher in stationary culture than in stirred culture (Table 1). Modifications to stirred culture that increase the productivity of these hybridoma lines two- to fourfold are only returning productivity to that found in stationary culture. Thus, trying the particular hybridoma line in the fantastic system is really the only way to obtain an accurate preduction of its productivity.

ACKNOWLEDGMENTS

The data reported in this chapter are the results of the efforts of and help from Joseph Gabriels, Julie Rudolph, Thomas Ducibella, Lucia van der Steur, Connie Gallop, and Lynne Rainen of Millipore Corp., and Monica Strzempko and Chris Cunningham of Hygeia Sciences.

REFERENCES

1. Kohler, G. and Milstein, C. (1975). Continuous cultures of fused cells secreting antibody of predefined specificity. *Nature 256*: 495–497.
2. Chandler, J. P. (1987). Factors influencing monoclonal antibody production in mouse ascites fluid. In *The Commercial Production of Monoclonal Antibodies.* Edited by S. S. Seaver. New York, Marcel Dekker, pp. 75–92.
3. de St. Groth, F. S. (1983). Automated production of monoclonal antibodies in a cytostat. *J. Immunol. Meth. 57*: 121–136.
4. Velez, D., Reuveny, S., Miller, L., and Macmillan, J. D. (1986). Kinetics of monoclonal antibody production in low serum growth medium. *J. Immunol. Meth. 86*: 45–52.
5. Lebherz, W. R. III. (1987). Batch production of monoclonal antibody by large-scale suspension cultures. In *The Commercial Production of Monoclonal Antibodies.* Edited by S. S. Seaver. New York, Marcel Dekker, pp. 93–118.
6. Arathoon, W. R. and Birch, J. R. (1986). Large-scale cell culture in biotechnology. *Science 232*: 1390–1395.
7. Hopkinson, J. (1985). Hollow fiber cell culture systems for economical cell-product manufacturing. *Bio/Technology 3*: 225–230.
8. Gruenberg, M. L., Tyo, M. A., and Potter, A. (1986). Optimization procedures for high density hybridoma cell cultures in Acusyst-P hollow fiber bioreactors. Presented at the Third Annual Congress for Automation, Scale-Up and the Economics of Biological Process Engineering, Baltimore, MD.
9. Brown, P. C., Costello, M., Oakley, R., and Lewis, J. (1985). Applications of mass culturing technique (MCT) in large-scale growth of mammalian cells. In *Large-Scale Mammalian Cell Culture.* Edited by J. Feder and W. R. Tolbert. New York, Academic Press, pp. 59–71.
10. Putnam, J. E. (1987). Monoclonal antibody production in a ceramic matrix. In *The Commercial Production of Monoclonal Antibodies.* Edited by S. S. Seaver. New York, Marcel Dekker, pp. 119–138.
11. Posillico, E. (1986). Microencapsulation technology for large scale antibody production. *Bio/Technology 4*: 114–117.
12. Seaver, S. S., Rudolph, J. L., and Gabriels, J. E. Jr. (1984). A rapid HPLC technique for monitoring amino acid utilization in cell culture. *Bio/Techniques 2*: 254–260.

13. Crespi, C. L., Imamura, I., Leong, P.-M., Fleischaker, R. J., Brunengraber, H., Thilly, W. G., and Giard, D. J. (1981). Microcarrier culture: Applications in biologicals production and cell biology. *Biotech. Bioeng. 23*: 2673-2689.
14. Reuveny, S., Velez, D., Macmillan, J. D., and Miller, L. (1986). Factors affecting cell growth and monoclonal antibody production in stirred reactors. *J. Immunol. Meth. 86*: 53-59.
15. McKeehan, W. L. (1982). Glycolysis, glutaminolysis and cell proliferation. *Cell Biol. Int. Rep. 6*: 635-650.
16. Gilbert, J. B., Price, V. E., and Greenstein, J. P. (1949). Effects of anions on the non-enzymatic disamidation of glutamine. *J. Biol. Chem. 180*: 209-218.
17. Wein, J. and Geotz, I. E. (1973). Asparginase and glutaminase activities in culture media containing dialyzed calf serum. *In Vitro 9*: 186-193.
18. McKeehan, W. L. and McKeehan, K. A. (1983). Alanine aminotransferase activity with unusually low glutamate and high pyruvate and alanine requirements in the cytosol of human fibroblasts. *In Vitro 19*: 255.
19. Chessebeuf, M., Mignot, G., and Padieu, P. (1983). Propagating rat liver epithelial cells on microcarriers either in serum-supplemented or in serum-free culture. *In Vitro 19*: 290.
20. Stoner, G. D. and Merchant, D. J. (1972). Amino acid utilization by L-M strain mouse cells in a chemically defined medium. *In Vitro 7*: 330-343.
21. Reuveny, S., Velez, D., Miller, L., and Macmillan, J. D. (1986). Comparison of cell propagation methods for their effect on monoclonal antibody yield in fermentors. *J. Immunol. Methods 86*: 61-69.
22. Seaver, S. S., Rudolph, J. L., Ducibells, T., and Gabriels, J. E. (1984). Hybridoma cell metabolism/antibody secretion in culture. In *World Biotech Report* 1984, Vol 2. New York, Online Publications, pp. 325-344.
23. Adamson, S. R., Behie, L. A., Gaucher, G. M., and Lesser, B. H. (1987). Metabolism of hybridoma cells in suspension culture: Evaluation of three commercially available media. In *The Commercial Production of Monoclonal Antibodies*. Edited by S. S. Seaver. New York, Marcel Dekker, pp. 17-34.
24. Brown, B. L. (1987). Reducing costs up front: A method for adapting myeloma and hybridoma cells to an inexpensive chemically defined serum-free medium. In *The Commercial Production of Monoclonal Antibodies*. Edited By S. S. Seaver. New York, Marcel Dekker, pp. 35-48.
25. Van Brunet, J. (1986). Immobilized mammalian cells: The gentle way to productivity. *Bio/Technology 4*: 505-510.

II
PRODUCTION IN LARGE-SCALE SYSTEMS

5

Factors Influencing Monoclonal Antibody Production in Mouse Ascites Fluid

JOSEPH P. CHANDLER*
Charles River Biotechnical Services, Inc., Wilmington, Massachusetts

I. INTRODUCTION

The development of hybridoma technology by Kohler and Milstein in 1975 (1) has provided a means of generating virtually unlimited quantities of antibodies. To produce monoclonal antibodies (MAb), the classic method has been by the injection of hybridoma cells into the peritoneal cavity of histocompatible mice (2,3), which, under appropriate conditions, results in formation of ascites. Ascites is a transudate (4,5) that forms in response to ascitogenic agents such as mineral oil, microorganisms, antigen–antibody complexes, and tumor cells. Most hybridoma cells, generated from the fusion of myeloma and spleen cells, are ascitogenic, and the ascites that forms during their peritoneal growth contains the MAb they secrete.

The successful implantation of hybridoma cells, the volume of ascites that can be collected from the peritoneal cavity, and the concentration of MAb/ unit volume of ascites are directly related to the biological behavior of the cell line. There are, however, a number of parameters under the control of the researcher. These factors become significantly important when the production scheme escalates from the generation of a few grams of MAb to large-scale MAb production in thousands of mice.

Charles River Biotechnical Services, Inc., (CRBS) has had the unique opportunity of handling large numbers of hybridoma cell lines through its contract in vivo MAb production service. It cannot be overemphasized that each cell line has behaved distinctly. The procedures established for the commercial

---

Present affiliation: Ventrex Laboratories, Inc., Portland, Maine.

production of MAbs by in vivo technology were designed to accommodate the individuality of each cell line while facilitating a routine production operation. As a result, any cell line, regardless of its idiosyncrasies, can be scaled-up to produce any amount of ascites without the need to "retool" the production system.

This chapter illustrates some of the characteristics of hybridoma cell lines defined by their in vivo growth characteristics and elaborates the steps in establishing a uniform production operation. The chapter will address those elements of commercial in vivo MAb production that can be manipulated to obtain maximum MAb output without recourse to further genetic manipulation of the cell line. These elements fall into two categories: standardization of mice and characterization of hybridoma cells.

II. STANDARDIZATION OF MICE

The optimal characteristics of mice that produce the most ascites have been defined through experiments and observation of certain trends as part of MAb production at CRBS and other laboratories. Each of these characteristics will be discussed below.

A. Pristane Priming of Mice

In early experiments, Cancro and Potter (6) and Hoogenraad and co-workers (7) found that ascites formation from the intraperitoneal (Ip) injection of plasmacytoma cells is dependent on preinjection of mineral oil or its pure alkane derivative, Pristane (2,6,10,14-tetramethylpentadecane). The preinjection of these irritants caused the influx of adherent cells that established a conditioned environment in the peritoneal cavity. Plasmacytoma cells established residence in this environment and thrived on the soluble growth factors secreted by the proliferating inflammatory cells. These studies suggested that Pristane pretreatment, or "priming," of mice should be a routine step in the ascites production operation.

An early study in this laboratory substantiated the need to prime mice with Pristane. In that experiment, 10-week-old female mice received an intraperitoneal injection of 1×10^5, 5×10^5, or 2×10^6 hybridoma cells. In none of these mice did ascites form. Solid tumors were found in some of the mice by 15 days following the injection of hybridoma cells. (Other groups of mice were given the same dosages of hybridoma cells but after a 3-week priming period. Ascites did develop in these mice; the results of that part of the experiment are shown in Table 3 and discussed later.) It appears from the reports in the literature and our experience that priming is essential to the successful growth of the hybridoma and to ascites formation.

However, in the course of the normal production operation, technicians have observed that even after priming some of the mice do not produce ascites as well as others. Postmortem examination of the mice has revealed that low ascites producers often had a few large masses of tumors growing in the peritoneal cavity, while high ascites producers have multiple small colonies of tumors growing extensively throughout the mesentery. In light of the work of Cancro and Potter (6), it could be suggested that the level of ascites formation is related to the granuloma formation resulting from the presence of the Pristane. At this writing, experimentation has not been performed to substantiate this claim; further investigation is warranted.

What has been defined, by analysis performed in the CRBS laboratory, is the time that should elapse between the Pristane priming of mice and the subsequent injection of hybridoma cells. Cancro and Potter (6) reported that a minimum of 3 days is required between Pristane priming and the injection of plasmacytoma cells to obtain successful cell growth and that a 30-day interval is optimal for maximum cell growth. Hoogenraad and colleagues (7) found that 10–20 days was optimal, while Brodeur et al. (8) reported that 14 days provided them with the best results.

Data obtained at CRBS on the scale-up production of two cell lines suggests that 3–4 weeks are required for maximum output of ascites. This is evident from the data presented in Figures 1 and 2. Figure 1 illustrates the results generated from cell line designated I, for which data were derived from the injection of 52 lots of male mice and 37 lots of female mice. Lots ranged in size from 200 to 1000 mice and all the mice were at least 10 weeks old. Priming periods ranged from 5 to 51 days. The relationship of the length of time between the priming of mice and the injection of hybridoma cells was plotted against the volume yield/mouse/lot. The data were subjected to linear regression analysis and segmented to generate a more exact curve. As can be seen, the yield of both male and female mice increased as the interval between priming and the injection of hybridoma cells increased. From 5 days to 20 days, the volume of ascites collected from male mice increased from 1.6 to 4.6 ml/mouse. After day 20, the volume continued to increase but less dramatically. For the female mice, the plateau did not occur until day 25.

Cell line II was also analyzed as above, but the data were based on 23 lots of male mice and 14 lots of female mice. Lot sizes ranged from 200 to 800 mice and the priming periods ranged from 5 to 54 days. The increase in the volume yields was found to be more gradual than that for cell line I. At the shorter priming period, the males were better producers of ascites than the female mice. The plateau for the males occurred after day 25. The female mice increased in ascites production with time and were comparable to the males after day 35.

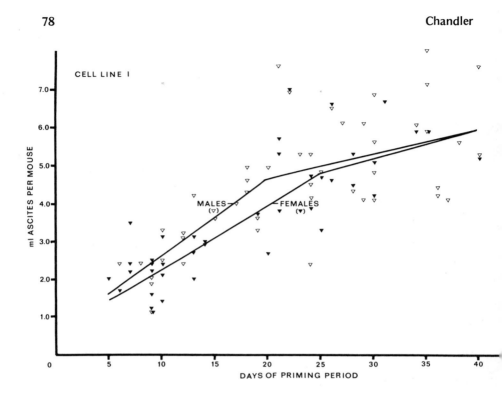

Figure 1   Increasing the length of time between the injection of Pristane into mice and the subsequent injection of hybridoma cells results in an increase in the volume of ascites collected per mouse. Mice were given 5×10^5 hybridoma cells of cell line I at various intervals after the intraperitoneal injection of Pristane and the ascites was collected three times. The volume of ascites per mouse was calculated by dividing the volume collected per lot by the number of mice injected. The regression curves determined from the male ($\triangledown$) and female ($\blacktriangledown$) data are delineated.

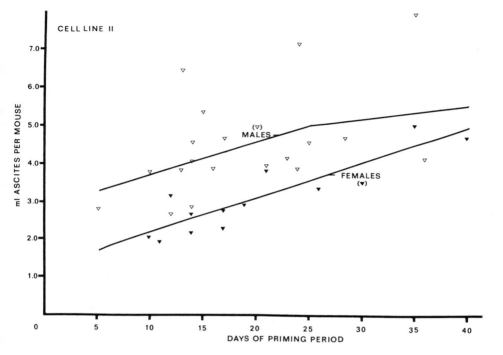

Figure 2   Increasing the length of time between the injection of Pristane into mice and the subsequent injection of hybridoma cells results in an increase in the volume of ascites collected per mouse. Mice were given 5×10^5 hybridoma cells of cell line II at various intervals after the intraperitoneal injection of Pristane and the ascites was collected three times. The volume of ascites per mouse was calculated by dividing the volume collected per lot by the number of mice injected. The regression curves determined from the male ($\triangledown$) and female ($\blacktriangledown$) data are delineated.

These data confirm that more than 3 weeks between the priming injection and the inoculation of hybridoma cells may be required to maximize the yields of ascites from a given lot of mice. It may be that the longer the priming period the more time the inflammatory cells have to establish conditions for hybridoma cell growth.

B. Strain of Mice

Almost all of the hybridoma cells received by this laboratory have been derived from BALB/c myeloma and spleen cells. They have been injected into BALB/c mice as standard procedure. A few cell lines were derivatives of BALB/c myeloma cells fused with C57BL/6 spleen cells. These were injected into the F1 hybrid of BALB/c $\times$ C57BL/6 mice, CB6 F1. The F1 hybrid was a successful ascites-producing mouse and was therefore considered a substitute for the parental strain.

An experiment was performed to compare the ascites generation of a BALB/c $\times$ BALB/c hybridoma in BALB/c mice and its F1 hybrids: the CB6 F1, CD2 F1 (BALB/c $\times$ DBA/2), and CD/c (CD1 outbred $\times$ BALB/c),* a strain bred for this experiment. The study was conducted in groups of 200 mice and each mouse was injected with 5×10^5 cells of an in-house-generated hybridoma cell line 25 days after being primed with Pristane. Ascites was collected sequentially in three "taps" (see below) and the percentage of mice tapped was determined as well as the volume of ascites collected and the milligrams of immunoglobulin/ml. As seen in Table 1, the cells grew successfully in all strains of mice and the results for each group were indistinguishable one from another and from the BALB/c mice. This work demonstrated that F1 hybrids can be used to produce ascites from a BALB/c parental cell line. However, the potential for a "stronger" mouse, which would allow for improved growth of hybridoma cells and ascites formation, is not substantiated by these data.

C. Sex of Mice

Scale-up production in mice has traditionally been performed in female retired-breeder mice due to a number of useful characteristics. They are often the largest mice available to a customer who does not want to wait for younger mice to mature. They are easy to handle and do not fight among themselves, as do the males. The aggressiveness of BALB/c males has been a significant deterrent to their use for any purpose. At CRBS we have

---

*These mice are not available for commercial sale.

Table 1   Ascites Production in BALB/c and BALB/c-F1 Hybrid Mice

Treatment group	Tap no.	% of Mice tappable	Volume collected	ml/Mouse	mg Ig/ml
CB6 F1	1	69.5	308[a]	2.2[b]	5.6
	2	67.0	306	2.2	7.8
	3	50.2	300	2.9	11.5
Total/average			914	5.0[c]	8.3
CD/c F1	1	75.3	350	2.5	3.0
	2	71.2	430	3.1	8.4
	3	41.4	254	2.5	12.2
Total/average			1034	5.4	7.5
CD2 F1	1	71.5	402	2.8	4.5
	2	59.5	340	2.8	7.8
	3	45.0	304	3.3	11.1
Total/average			1046	5.3	7.5
BALB/c	1	86.7	485	2.8	4.1
	2	77.5	378	2.4	8.3
	3	48.6	223	2.3	11.6
Total/average			1086	5.4	7.1

Ascites was generated by inoculating each group of 200 mice intraperitoneally with 5×10^5 hybridoma cells 25 days after Pristane priming. Ascites was collected three times starting on day 12 after the injection of cells.
[a]Volume measured after centrifugation.
[b]Volume/number of mice tapped.
[c]Volume/number of mice injected.

minimized male aggression through a number of techniques, such as housing males together from the time they are weaned.

Strictly in terms of capacity of ascites production, we have not, in general, found one sex better than the other. A specific cell line may grow slightly better in one sex than in the other, but this preference cannot be forecasted. When a difference is observed, it is in the percentage of mice that can be tapped, not in the volume of ascites collected per mouse. With some cell lines, solid tumors tend to form in one sex while normal ascites forms in the other. Again, this is not predictable, nor is it prevalent in one sex over the other. It appears to be dependent upon the inherent behavior of the cell line.

D. "Tapping" of Mice

One factor that can significantly affect the volume of ascites and the total MAb harvested is the method used to collect the ascites. The method employed in this laboratory is a sequential harvesting technique we have dubbed "tapping," which experiments have shown superior to a single-harvest method (see Tables 2 and 3). Most laboratories use one of these two methods. In single-harvest, the mice are euthanized, their peritoneal cavity is exposed, and the ascites aspirated from the cavity. In tapping, one technique is to hold the live animal, insert a syringe needle (about 18 g), and let the ascites drip out by natural pressure.

At CRBS, gentle aspiration of ascites from the live mouse is preferred as the most thorough and the least traumatic for the animal. In this technique, a collection flask is connected to a vacuum pump. A needle is attached to sterile tubing, which is connected to the flask and inserted into the peritoneal cavity. With a little dexterity and practice, ascites begins to flow into the flask. The system allows for rapid, thorough, and aseptic ascites collection, which is particularly important when hundreds of mice need to be tapped daily.

Our early experiment indicated that sequential tapping would provide the highest yields of ascites and the greatest concentrations of MAb from a given lot of mice. This finding was confirmed by experiments performed when we were developing our production service. Table 2 illustrates the results obtained from two experiments in which BALB/c mice were given 1×10^6 hybridoma cells 14 days following injection of Pristane. The hybridoma secreted an antibody with specificity to sheep red blood cells. The mice were tapped at days 14, 17, and 20 after the injection of hybridoma cells. As can be seen, excellent yields of ascites were obtained from both groups of mice. In the first experiment, 143 ml ascites was collected from 16 mice (8.9 ml/mouse injected) and 260 ml was collected from 30 mice (8.6 ml/mouse injected). In each tap, high concentrations of antibody were present as

Table 2 Change in Monoclonal Antibody (MAb) Titers in Consecutive
Collections of Ascites (Taps)

Tap no.	Number of mice tapped	Volume (ml) collected	MAb titer
Experiment 1			
1	6/16[a]	27 (4.5)[b]	1:12,800
2	14/14	74 (5.3)	1:25,600
3	8/8	42 (5.2)	1:25,600
Total		143 (8.9)	
Experiment 2			
1	29/30	105 (3.6)	1:16,000
2	25/26	129 (5.1)	1:32,000
3	6/7	26 (4.3)	1:32,000
Total		260 (8.6)	

Mice were inoculated intraperitoneally with 1×10^6 hybridoma cells 14 days after Pristane priming. The mice were tapped three times and the anti-sheep red blood cell antibody in the ascites was detected in a hemagglutination assay.
[a]Volume measured after centrifugation.
[b]Value in parentheses is ml/mouse.

evident by the high antibody titer (as determined by a standard hemagglutination assay performed in V-bottomed microtiter plates).

As the experiment progressed, fewer mice were available for tapping since mice died from growth of the hybridoma. Subsequent experiments were performed to determine the best dosage of cells, that is, the concentration of cells that would grow in the highest percentage of mice injected but allow for maximum animal survival. As shown in Table 3, high, medium, and low dosages of a hybridoma cell line were injected into groups of 20 BALB/c mice, and the ascites was collected between days 14 to 25 depending on the rate of ascites development. The greatest percentage of mice to develop ascites occurred in the group receiving the highest dosage (20/20), but half of the mice had died by the second tap. In the medium-dosage group, most of the animals developed ascites and greater than half of the mice were still alive by the third tap. In the low-dosage group, fewer mice developed ascites and the volume yields collected per mouse at a tap were considerably less than in the other two groups. The group receiving 5×10^5 produced

Table 3   Ascites Produced in BALB/c Mice Inoculated with Different Doses of Hybridoma Cells

Cells no.	Tap no.	Number of mice tapped	Volume (ml) collected	Volume ml/mouse
1×10^5	1	10/19[a]	33	3.3
	2	14/19	47	3.3
	3	14/19	34	2.4
			(114)[b]	(6.0)[c]
5×10^5	1	17/19	86	5.0
	2	17/18	93	5.5
	3	14/15	54	3.8
			(233)	(12.2)
2×10^6	1	20/20	98	4.9
	2	9/9	40	4.5
	3	4/4	12	3.0
			(150)	(7.5)

Mice were inoculated intraperitoneally with different dosages of hybridoma cells and tapped three times.
[a]Number of mice tapped/number of mice remaining alive.
[b]Total volume of ascites collected.
[c]Average ml/mouse collected/number of mice injected.

the greatest total yield of ascites and had a consistently higher yield of ascites per mouse per tap. The volume collected from a mouse is often dependent upon the hybridoma cell line (to be discussed later) but the results of this experiment were typical; they led us to use 5×10^5 cells as a standard inoculum for the scale-up operation.

The decision to perform sequential collection of ascites was also based on the finding that MAb concentration increased with each successive tap. Tables 4 and 5 show the results of two similarly performed experiments. In these studies, groups of 20 mice were inoculated with different dosages of hybridoma cells 21 days after Pristane priming and they were tapped between 14 and 25 days depending on the rate of ascites development for the group. In the first experiment, mice were inoculated with hybridoma cells that

Table 4   Monoclonal Antibody[a] (MAb)
Titers in Ascites Generated with Different
Doses of Cells: Experiment 1

No. of cells	Tap no.	MAb titer
1×10^5	1	1: 2,000
	2	1: 32,000
	3	1: 64,000
5×10^5	1	1: 4,000
	2	1: 32,000
	3	1:256,000
2×10^6	1	1: 16,000
	2	1:128,000
	3	1:128,000

Mice were inoculated intraperitoneally with different doses of hybridoma cells 21 days after Pristane priming. The mice were tapped three times
and the antibody titer was determined by a
hemagglutination assay.
[a]IgM with specificity to sheep red cells.

secreted an IgG with specificity for sheep red blood cells; in the second, the
antibody was an IgM with the same specificity. As can be seen, antibody
titers increased from the first tap to the third. The dosage of cells given to
the mice did not appear to be a major factor in the antibody titer. (The
difference between titers must be more than twofold to be considered significantly different.) It is considered important, therefore, to tap mice more
than once since the amount of MAb collected is greatest after a number of
taps are performed. (Taps need not be limited to three. This is the practice
at CRBS because with most cell lines only 10–25% of the mice survive to the
third tap. There are, however, a few cell lines that do not kill the mice so
rapidly.)

Production results have also demonstrated the value of successive tapping.
Table 6 shows a few cell lines that have been processed in this laboratory.
In each case, immunoglobulin (Ig) concentration increased with each tap.
(The Ig concentrations reported in Table 6 were calculated from the percent

Table 5 Monoclonal Antibody[a] (MAb) Titer in Ascites Generated with Different Doses of Cells: Experiment 2

No. of cells	Tap no.	MAb titer
1×10^5	1	1: 2,000
	2	1:16,000
	3	1:64,000
5×10^5	1	1: 4,000
	2	1:16,000
	3	1:32,000
2×10^6	1	1: 8,000
	2	1:32,000
	3[b]	—

Mice were inoculated intraperitoneally with different doses of hybridoma cell 21 days after Pristane priming. The mice were tapped three times and the antibody titer was determined by an hemagglutination assay.
[a]IgG with specificity to sheep red cells.
[b]All mice died prior to tapping.

Table 6 Increasing Immunoglobulin (Ig) Concentration in Successive "Taps"

Cell line	mg Ig/ml ascites		
	Tap 1	Tap 2	Tap 3
H	3.1	4.3	4.4
W	2.4	3.8	5.3
B	3.0	5.7	6.1
V	3.4	5.2	6.7
U	1.4	6.6	7.4
G	5.1	9.5	12.4
N	7.5	12.7	13.3
L	4.8	11.4	15.3
T	8.9	23.0	26.0

Mice were inoculated intraperitoneally with contract hybridoma cells. The concentration of Ig was determined by cellulose acetate electrophoresis.

of Ig, as detected by cellulose acetate electrophoresis [CAE],* multiplied by the total protein of the ascites as measured by biuret analysis.) Of particular interest is the range of MAb concentrations that can be obtained with different cell lines (discussed below). What contributes to the final concentration in a lot of ascites, of course, is the concentration of MAb per tap and the portion that each tap contributes to the final pool of ascites.

III. CHARACTERIZATION OF HYBRIDOMA CELLS

As a contract producer of MAb, CRBS has found that once a given cell line successfully grows in mice little can be done to increase its production. Production capacity is largely a genetic trait, and "improvements" will come from advances made by genetic engineers. However, for the purposes of this discussion, two subjects will be broached: the adaptation of cell lines to in vivo growth, and the range of results encountered by the cell lines grown in mice in this laboratory.

A. Adaptation of Hybridoma Cell Lines to In Vivo Growth

Start-up production can sometimes be impeded by cell line variation over which the researcher has considerable control. Once a cell line has been generated, for example, it may not grow readily in mice. This is not unusual and can be remedied. If a group of mice is injected with cells and none of the mice develop ascites, there are ways of adapting cells to in vivo growth.

One method is to inject a few mice intradermally with 1-5 $\times$ 10^6 cell. Most cell lines will grow at this site. Once there is a sizable tumor (not too large since tumors at this site tend to ulcerate), the mass can be aseptically removed and mechanically or enzymatically disrupted to produce a single cell suspension. This pool of cells can be used to inoculate a culture and another group of primed mice that should, in turn, develop ascites.

The next technique is useful when a group of mice is injected and only some of them develop ascites. In this procedure, animals are given an Ip injection of 1-5 $\times$ 10^6 cells 3-4 weeks following Pristane priming. Those which begin to show signs of ascites formation become the source of cells for further passage of the line. Their cells are collected by lavage of the peritoneal cavity using sterile physiological saline. The cells are cultivated in vitro and reinjected into a new group of primed mice. (For both of these

---

*This is performed using Helena Laboratory products. The ascites is applied to Titan III plates and subjected to electrophoresis at 200 mV for 20-30 min. The plates are stained with Ponseau S, clarified, and read in a Quik Scan Jr. densitometer.

techniques, the number of in vivo passages should be limited since natural selection can modify the cell line to produce a new population of cells that could secrete a variant MAb or, worse yet, none at all.)

In this laboratory, a pilot study is performed by inoculating newly acquired hybridoma cells into a few mice to discover any peculiar in vivo growth characteristics. Once the general growth behavior of the cell line has been determined, scale-up can be performed more successfully. A number of cell lines have been adapted for in vivo growth without alterations in the antibody-secreting characteristic.

B. Hybridoma Cell Line Characteristics

As mentioned, the MAb production factor that cannot be readily controlled is the biological behavior of the cell line. Attempts can be made to moderate the behavior of the cells by optimizing the mice to be injected, but the basic capacity for the production of ascites—its volume and concentration of antibody—is directly dependent on the characteristics of the cell line.

Table 7 shows the range of results obtained in this laboratory with different cell lines. The cell lines are listed in order of increasing MAb concentration, as determined by first performing CAE on the ascites and obtaining the percentage Ig by reading the clarified plates in a densitometer. The mg/ml protein was then determined by the biuret technique and the mg/ml immunoglobulin was calculated from these data. The table lists some of the cell lines we have processed. The data represent results obtained from a lot of mice with a given cell line or the mean of the lots, if more than one lot of ascites was generated by the line.

At this writing, CRBS has produced more than 3.3 kg antibody contained in slightly over 460 L ascites. The average MAb concentration in ascites is 6.9 mg Ig/ml and 4.8 ml/mouse for ascites production. There is a broad range of results, as shown in Table 7, with the most productive cell line producing nearly 7.5 times the MAb concentration of the least productive. The volumes of ascites per lot ranges less broadly than MAb concentrations, with a 3.5-fold difference between the most productive (8.4 ml/mouse) and the least productive (2.4 ml/mouse).

If the comparison of cell lines is extended to include the amount of Ig/mouse, the range is again quite large. For example, cell line P would only yield 8 mg Ig/mouse, while cell line A would yield 116 mg. In scale-up terms, this means that 1 g antibody could be obtained from as few as 9 mice for cell line A but 125 mice would be needed for cell line P. Some cell lines can yield large amounts of antibody in relatively few mice. While most cell lines probably fall into the range seen here, greater MAb-producing cell lines may become more common with greater use of genetic engineering.

Table 7 Volume and MAb Yields in Lots of Ascites Generated by Different Cell Lines

Cell line	ml/Mouse[a,b]	mg Ig/ml[b]	mg Ig/mouse[c]
AA	4.7	1.8	8.4
DD	5.0	1.8	9.0
P	4.0	2.0	8.0
NN	5.0	2.4	12.0
K	3.6	2.7	9.7
BB	5.5	2.8	15.4
LL	4.9	2.9	14.2
J	3.1	3.3	10.2
E	5.6	3.5	19.6
W	6.4	3.5	22.4
H	3.4	3.8	12.9
B	4.5	4.0	18.0
Z	3.8	4.1	15.6
V	4.2	4.1	17.2
JJ	4.3	4.3	18.5
KK	6.1	4.4	26.8
U	3.9	5.0	19.5
HH	3.5	5.4	18.9
MM	3.9	5.7	22.2
X	3.4	6.2	21.1
CC	4.6	6.9	31.7
GG	4.2	7.4	31.1
T	2.4	7.5	18.0
Y	4.4	7.5	33.0
D	7.2	7.8	51.8
II	3.8	8.0	30.4
L	4.8	8.0	38.4
EE	3.8	8.1	30.8
G	14.1	8.1	114.2
I	5.5	9.0	49.5
Q	4.5	9.1	40.9

Table 7   (Continued)

Cell line	ml/Mouse[a,b]	mg Ig/ml[b]	mg Ig/mouse[c]
N	4.9	9.6	47.0
FF	5.9	9.6	56.6
O	4.3	10.0	43.0
M	4.3	10.8	46.4
R	4.2	13.3	55.8
A	8.4	13.4	115.9

Mice were inoculated intraperitoneally with contract hybridoma cells. Ig concentration was determined by cellulose acetate electrophoresis.
[a]ml/Mouse injected.
[b]Average of lot or lots of mice injected.
[c]ml/Mouse × mg Ig/ml ascites.

Table 8   Range of Ascites and MAb Yields Observed from Different Lot of Mice Injected With the Same Cell Line

Cell line	ml/Mouse	mg/ml
E	6.4–7.1	3.5– 4.0
T	2.0–2.8	7.3– 7.8
B	4.1–6.3	2.9– 6.3
A	5.0–9.1	11.6–17.3
N	2.3–6.8	8.8–10.5
G	1.7–7.6	4.1–17.0
L	2.4–8.6	3.8–13.4

Mice were inoculated intraperitoneally with contract hybridoma cells. Ig concentration was determined by cellulose acetate electrophoresis.

It would appear that the volume of ascites collected from mice injected with a cell line may be as much a characteristic of that cell line as the concentration of MAb secreted. As discussed in the section on Pristane priming, the controlling factor in the volume yields could be related to the manner of the tumor growth within the peritoneal cavity.

It would also appear that lot-to-lot variation of yield (both the volume of ascites and MAb concentration) is characteristic of a given cell line. As mentioned above, Table 7 represents the mean yield for many of the cell lines processed by this laboratory. In Table 8, fluctuations among lots of mice injected with the same cell line are shown. (A number of requests for ascites have required the injection of more than one lot of mice to produce the needed quantity of MAb.) According to these results, it seemed characteristic that some lines are subject to little fluctuation, while others fluctuate dramatically from lot to lot. Significant efforts have been made in this laboratory to moderate cell line behavior and minimize lot-to-lot variation, for example, by using the same sex and similar age for different lots. We recognize, of course, that variation is not due solely to the cells but also to a number of human factors. The researcher does, however, have limited control over lot-to-lot variation, as noted throughout this chapter.

IV. CONCLUSION

We have attempted to describe the many variables that this laboratory has observed and analyzed as pertinent to the generation of MAb-rich ascites. For those variables analyzed in controlled experiments, we have defined rationale. It becomes increasingly more difficult to account for every variation observed in production runs, but we have discussed certain trends that seem readily apparent.

The surest way to achieve maximum ascites production and MAb yields would be to screen the original clones in mice and to use the one providing the best results. When this is not feasible—and for many hybridomas it may not be—the best approach is to use mice that can best produce ascites. This chapter offers a profile of these animals based on the experience of CRBS and others working in large-scale MAb production.

REFERENCES

1. Kohler, G. and Milstein, C. (1975). Continuous culture of fused cells secreting antibody of defined specificity. *Nature 256*: 495–497.
2. Kennett, R. J., McKearn, T. J., and Bechtol, K. B. (eds.). (1980). *Monoclonal Antibodies—Hybridomas: A New Dimension in Biological Analyses*. New York, Plenum Press.

3. Langone, J. J. and van Vunakis, H. (eds.). (1983). *Methods in Enzymology. Vol. 92 Immunochemical Techniques Part E Monoclonal Antibodies and General Immunoassay Methods.* New York, Academic Press.
4. Duncan, J. R. and Prasse, K. W. (eds.). (1977). *Veterinary Laboratory Medicine—Clinical Pathology.* Ames, Iowa, Iowa State University Press.
5. Jones, C. J. and Hunt, R. D. (eds.). (1983). *Veterinary Pathology*, 5th edition. Philadelphia, Lea & Febiger.
6. Cancro, M. and Potter, M. (1976). The requirement of an adherent cell substratum for the growth of developing plasmacytoma cell in vivo. *J. Exp. Med. 144*: 1554–1567.
7. Hoogenraad, N., Helman, T., and Hoogenraad, J. (1983). The effect of pre-injection of mice with Pristane on ascites tumour formation and monoclonal antibody production. *J. Immunol. Methods 61*: 317–320.
8. Brodeur, B. R., Tsang, P., and Larose, Y. (1985). Parameters affecting ascites tumour formation in mice and monoclonal antibody production. *J. Immunol. Methods 71*: 265–272.

6

Batch Production of Monoclonal Antibody by Large-Scale Suspension Culture

WILLIAM B. LEBHERZ III
Program Resources, Inc., National Cancer Institute–Frederick Cancer Research Facility, National Institutes of Health, Frederick, Maryland

I. INTRODUCTION

In the 10 years since Kohler and Milstein (1,2) first reported their work on the development of hybridomas, the scientific world has seen a rapid adaptation of this technique and an expansion of its usefulness not unlike that which followed the discovery of antibiotics (3). Applications of hybridoma methodology show a diversity far beyond that envisioned by its originators. These "engineered" bioactive proteins have entered such fields as agriculture, biochemistry, diagnostics, medicine, microbiology, pharmaceutics, and virology. More recently, the field of law has even been affected as designers of these cell systems obtain patents on their "inventions."

The products of these hybridomas—monoclonal antibodies—are expected to play a significant role in the field of cancer diagnosis and therapy (4-6). Monoclonal antibodies constructed against human tumor-associated antigens used either alone or coupled to radiotracers or a variety of cytotoxic materials are current conceptual models enjoying the attention of the medical community. Several are currently undergoing phase I clinical trials either as treatments in and of themselves or as diagnostic tools (7).

The traditional method for producing monoclonal antibodies is by intraperitoneal injection of the hybridoma cells into pristane-primed syngeneic mice or other suitable hosts. Another method is by production of large amounts of conditioned medium in which hybridomas capable of secreting the antibody are grown (8).

In 1982 this facility became involved in production of gram quantities of highly purified monoclonal antibody from cell cultures. This material was to be produced under the conditions of current Good Manufacturing Practices (GMPs) and was to be provided to the Biological Response Modifiers Program (BRMP) operated by the NCI Division of Cancer Treatment. The task of this facility was to manufacture the antibody as a bulk sterile product. Final finishing of the monoclonal antibody was to be performed at other government-contracted facilities.

This chapter discusses our experiences in setting up and routinely operating a manufacturing area for producing highly pure monoclonal antibody from submerged hybridoma cultures grown in stainless steel fermentors. Some general attention will be given to the methods used to purify the antibody but persons specifically interested in this aspect are directed to read Chapter 11, Affinity Purification of Monoclonal Antibody From Tissue Culture Supernatant Using Protein A-Sepharose CL-4B, by Dr. Shwu-Maan Lee.

II. THE MANUFACTURING ENTITY

In conceptualizing this task we first looked upon the hybridoma as an entity unto itself. Our early studies were therefore designed to understand this entity and, in a sense, let it teach us its needs and capabilities. Our production models were then based on this knowledge.

A. Creating and Characterizing the Hybridoma

The 9.2.27 hybridoma, developed and characterized by Dr. A. C. Morgan, Jr., and two co-workers in 1981 (9), produces a murine IgG_{2a} that recognizes a melanoma-specific 250 K dalton glycoprotein/proteoglycan. This particular antigen has been observed in spent melanoma-cell-conditioned medium or on the surface of melanoma cells (10).

The antibody produced by the 9.2.27 hybridoma has a molecular weight of 150,000 daltons. In our cell culture system the hybridoma has a doubling time of 9–15 hr and usually maintains a viability of 90–95% during the exponential phase of growth.

In 1982 this antibody–antigen model was being considered as a candidate for phase I clinical trials by the BRMP. Although sufficient amounts of antibody for research and development were being recovered from conditioned medium from multiple T-flasks or roller bottles and from ascites, it was evident that larger amounts of material would be required for the variety of studies routinely required for potential new drugs. We were provided with a T-flask culture of this hybridoma with the directive that a suspension culture system be developed and optimized for producing large quantities of highly purified antibody. While a body of literature existed regarding the growth of mammalian cells in large-scale systems (11,12) there was, at that time, little information on the growth of hybridomas in fermentors (13). Our initial approach had several objectives. These were to (a) develop and define parameters for a suspension culture system in glass vessels, with later scale-up into 50 L fermentors; (b) determine the best culture milieu for the hybridoma based upon antibody productivity, economics and quality of product; and (c) determine the best method for recovering the antibody in a highly pure form.

Since the cell culture was originally provided to our laboratory as a "static" suspension culture, the first step was adaptation of the culture to growth in spinner flasks. First attempts at growing the 9.2.27 hybridoma in conventional 100 ml spinner flasks revealed that the culture could be managed in a manner similar to routine procedures we had applied to most suspension cultures in our production facilities. That is, the culture could easily be maintained in the log phase of growth by ensuring that the inoculation density was kept within a range that ensured consistent and reproducible population doubling times. For this hybridoma the range was $4-8 \times 10^4$ viable cells (vc) per ml. Transfers were performed at densities between 1 and 2×10^6 vc/ml. Dulbeccos' Modified Eagle Medium (DMEM) was used in these preliminary studies. Antibiotics were never used in maintenance, scale-up, or production medium formulations. Subsequent experiments utilized varied levels of fetal calf serum (FCS) to determine the effects on cell growth. As expected, we observed (data not shown) a reduction in doubling time and a decrease in upper log phase density with decreased levels of serum.

Following the development of a suitable assay (ELISA) for the antibody in cell culture samples (14), we then examined other medium formulations and repeated a comparison of various serum levels in DMEM to discern the kinetics of antibody release. Repeated experiments in spinner flasks containing DMEM with 5% and 3% FCS showed that the antibody reached its peak in the culture medium at 24-72 hr after the saturation density had been reached and during the death phase of the culture (Fig. 1). Subsequent experiments with various formulations of commercially available culture medium or serum substitutes purported to be especially good for the growth of hybridomas showed a similar but not better production profile. The three best formulations as determined by peak antibody titer were then compared as to cost/10 L of medium. Results are shown in Table 1. Dulbecco's Modified Eagle Medium was selected as the production medium on the basis of this comparison.

In summary, preliminary studies indicated that the cells would grow in conventional glass spinners as true suspension cultures in an easily obtainable commercial medium and, when supplemented with 2-10% FCS, would produce

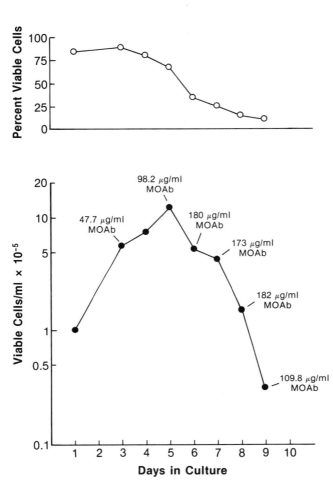

Figure 1 Comparison of cell growth, viability, and titer of 9.2.27 monoclonal antibody. Open circles, percent viability; closed circles, viable cells/ml. Cells were grown in 100 ml glass spinners in DMEM plus 5% fetal calf serum. MOAb, monoclonal antibody.

Table 1   Comparison of Costs, Native Protein Level, and Antibody Titers
Obtained with Four Medium Formulations[a]

Type of medium	Cost/10 L[b]	Protein level (mg/ml)	Antibody titer[c] (μg/ml)
DMEM + 3% FCS	$ 29.10	2.92	160
DMEM + 5% NU Serum[d]	$ 52.17	1.78	107
HSI-LoSM + 1.25% FCS[e]	$ 98.30	1.3	114.5
HB101 w/o Serum[f]	$183.30	1.98	ND[g]

[a]Cell cultures were grown in 100 ml glass spinners.
[b]Cost is in 1982 dollars.
[c]As determined by ELISA.
[d]NU serum is a serum substitute marketed by Collaborative Research, Inc.
[e]HSI-LoSM is a low serum-containing medium marketed by Hybridoma Sciences, Inc. It
was supplemented with 1.25% fetal calf serum.
[f]HB101 is a serum-free medium manufactured by HANA Media, Inc. and marketed by
NEN Products.
[g]ND, not done.

significant amounts of antibody (Table 2) at a reasonable cost. The next
step was to introduce the cells to stirred, controlled reactors and to develop
a model for production in 50 L fermentors.

B. Developing Production Models

Since initial studies had been performed in 100 ml glass spinner flasks, the
cultures were advanced to 500 ml spinner flasks. These trials, using DMEM
plus 3% FCS, resulted in greater concentrations of secreted antibody in the
larger vessel (Table 3). Presumably, the larger flask presented a more bene-
ficial environment (geometry) to these cells.

   In an effort to understand better the performance of these cells in larger
vessels with more controlled environments the cultures were introduced into
14 L stir jars (Chemapec, Inc.) that had been modified in our laboratories for
cell culture. These units provided an opportunity to control and record
several parameters known or assumed to effect growth rates and/or productivity. These were pH, dissolved oxygen, and agitation rate. Again, with
the use of DMEM plus 3% FCS, the cells grew and produced antibody similar
in pattern to that seen in glass spinners (Table 4). One observable difference
was that the death rate, during which relatively large amounts of antibody
are released into the medium, was considerably slower than that observed in

Table 2 Comparison of Antibody Titers and Specific Activity
with Serum Level[a]

Percent serum (volume/volume)	Antibody titer[b] (μg/ml)	Specific activity (μg/mg total protein)
2	72	150
3	67	84
5	120	75
10	170	58

[a]Comparisons were performed in 100 ml spinner flasks with DMEM.
[b]Antibody titer as determined by ELISA. Values represent the highest titer
observed during the culture period.

conventional spinners (data not shown). This is presumed to be due to the
more highly controlled environment presented in the stir jar.

Based on these studies it was now possible to construct a batch production
model in large stirred vessels with the potential for producing large quantities
of conditioned medium containing the antibody at levels acceptable for our
recovery methods (60–120 μg/ml). Although serum had been used at levels
ranging from 2 to 10% in DMEM, the highest titers had been achieved at
5–10% (refer to Table 2). This fact, coupled with a unique one-step purification procedure developed by Dr. Shwu-Maan Lee and others at the NCI-FCRF
(15; Chap. 11) led our group to propose using DMEM plus 10% FCS in all

Table 3 Effect of Scale-Up on Antibody Levels at Three
Time Points[a]

Nominal spinner volume (ml)	Antibody levels[b] (μg/ml)		
	48 hr[c]	96 hr	144 hr
100	10 (ND)[d]	51 (64)	67 (84)
500	33 (41)	79 (105)	160 (205)

[a]Cultures were grown in DMEM plus 3% fetal calf serum.
[b]Antibody titers were determined by ELISA. Values in parentheses
are specific activity in μg antibody/mg total protein.
[c]Times are hours of culture at which samples were obtained.
[d]ND, not done.

Table 4 Production of 9.2.27 Monoclonal Antibody in 14 L Stir Jars[a]

Time in culture (hr)	Antibody titer (μg/ml)[b]		
	Run[c] 1	Run 2	Run 3
70	105	105	41
120	130	145	163
168	ND[d]	135	135

[a]All cultures were grown in 14 L stir jars with a 10 L working volume. The stir jars were obtained from Chemapec, Inc. in Woodbury, N.Y. These were trial runs set up to assess the response of cells grown under more controlled environments and at volumes larger than conventional spinner flasks.
[b]Antibody levels were determined by ELISA.
[c]Runs 1 and 2 used DMEM + 3% fetal calf serum. Run 3 used DMEM + 5% NU serum.
[d]ND, not done.

maintenance and scale-up cultures with a stepwise decrease to DMEM + 7% FCS in the cell culture fermentor.

III. MANUFACTURING ENVIRONMENT

We look upon the manufacturing environment as composed of three inter-related components. These are the physical plant, the hardware or equipment, and the people. The role and relationship of each needed to be clearly defined to produce a manageable manufacturing process in a short period of time (4–5 months).

A. Physical Plant

The production area layout is shown in Figure 2. This area is sandwiched between two other areas involved in prokaryotic production and research and development. For this reason, an air lock was installed at the entrance into the antibody production area and the overall air balance within the area was positive in a gradient moving from the labs (rooms 9 and 10) and the fermentor room (room 12) into the hallway and then towards outside areas. The other doors shown in the diagram are for emergency exit only. Production, purification, and preparation of sterile bulk product were performed in this area.

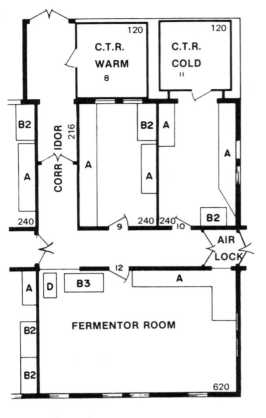

Room 9
   ELISA Assay Area
   Sample Processing
   Glassware Preparation

Room 10
   Seed Maintenance and
     Scale-Up
   Sterile Filtration of
     Final Product
   Antibody Purification
     (cold room)

Room 12
   Production Area
   Cell Removal
   Antibody Concentration

Legend

A = Workbench
B2 = Laminar Flow Hood
B3 = Class 1 Hood
D = Autoclave

Figure 2 Production area design. Small numbers in the corner of each room are square feet. Room numbers are shown in the entrances to each room. C.T.R., constant temperature room. Entrance is through the air lock.

To be in compliance with GMPs, several modifications had to be made to the production area. Continuous seamless flooring was installed in each lab and in the hallways but not in the fermentor room, which had a painted concrete floor. Non-particle-shedding ceiling tiles were installed throughout the area. The fermentor room had its own air supply while the hallway and labs were supported by a separate system. Water supply was of three types: tap, reverse osmosis deionized (RODI), and depyrogenated (ultrafiltered). The tap and RODI water lines were available in each lab and in the fermentor room. The depyrogenated water was generated in the fermentor room from a point-of-use ultrafiltration unit (Hydro-Services, Inc.) fed with RODI water. The depyrogenated water was used as make-up water for all buffers, fermentor medium, and other product contact reagents. It was also used as a final rinse for fermentors, process lines, equipment, glassware, etc. The waters were routinely monitored by the Quality Control (QC) unit for acceptability regarding pH, conductivity, and oxidizable substances. Less frequent monitoring of work stations or process points for bioburden and pyrogen level was performed by the Quality Assurance (QA) unit. The constant temperature rooms (CTR) were painted and disinfected prior to dedication of the area. Entrance was limited to those persons with responsibility for the production of the 9.2.27 antibody. Workers were required to wear fresh scrub suits or disposable surgeons' gowns, nurses' caps, shoe covers, and, when engaged in processing, disposable gloves.

B. Hardware

Cell culture maintenance and scale-up was performed in standard glass spinner flasks (Bellco, 1969 series).

Cell counts were performed in hemacytometers using a dye-exclusion method for assessment of viability. Large-scale production was performed in eight 50 L fermentors (New Brunswick Scientific Co.). Parameters under automatic or operator-initiated control included pH, dissolved oxygen, aeration rate, temperature, and agitation rate. The basic fermentor design, operating parameters, and culture medium components are shown in Figure 3.

Cells were removed via continuous flow centrifugation in an Alfa-Laval centrifuge. Supernatant was then pooled and held at 2-8°C in a jacketed stainless steel tank designed and constructed in-house. Concentration of antibody in the supernatant was performed with a stainless steel Pellicon (Millipore Corp.) fitted with 100,000 dalton nominal molecular weight cut-off polysulfone membranes. Antibody was adsorbed from the concentrated supernatant in a Pharmacia K100/45 column containing 150 g (dry weight) of protein A-Sepharose CL-4B (Pharmacia). A precolumn (Glenco) containing approximately 200 ml Sepharose CL-4B was placed in line prior to the protein

A. **Fermentor Design**

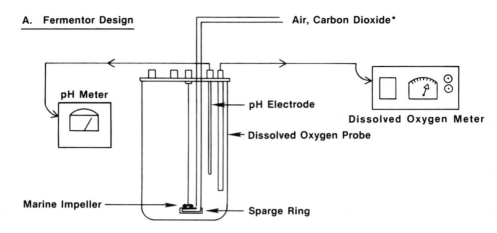

*Venting mechanisms, pressure regulating system, heating/cooling systems not shown.

B. **Operating Parameters**

Temperature	$37 \pm 0.5°C$
Agitation rate (tip speed)	100 rpm (4000 cm/min)
pH Range	7.0 ± 0.3
Dissolved oxygen	>10% saturation
Pressure (head-space)	5 ± 3 psig
Working volume/total volume	35/50 L

C. **Culture Medium**

DMEM (powder) with 4500 mg D-glucose/L	13.37 g/L
Fetal bovine serum	7% (v/v)
Sodium pyruvate	100 mg/L
HEPES buffer	10 mM
L-Glutamine	4 mM
Sodium bicarbonate	3.7 g/L

Figure 3 Basic fermentor design, operating parameters, and culture medium. Shown is a 50 L New Brunswick Tissue Culture fermentor. Dissolved oxygen was measured by a polaragraphic probe (Ingold Electrodes, Inc.) and pH was measured by an Ingold pH probe in a pressurizable housing. Medium was made up in a stainless steel tank and filtered through 0.22 μm hydrophilic filters (Pall Trincor Corp.) and into the sterile fermentor.

A column to prevent fouling of the affinity column. The flow rate of 52 cm/hr produced an operating pressure of 0.25 bar.

Final concentration of the column eluent fractions was performed with the Pellicon unit referred to previously. After formulation, the concentrated antibody was sterile filled into 500 ml serum bottles through a 0.22 μm Sealkleen filter (Pall Trincor Corporation).

C. Staffing

Three separate groups interacted very closely in this production campaign: the production unit, the QA unit, and the QC unit. The production unit, as its name implies, was responsible for all aspects of production from the initiation of seed to the sterile filling of bulk product. This group of six persons include a production manager, a plant foreman, two plant operators, a purification technician, and a cell culturist. The cell culturist managed the cells in a lab environment up to the generation of 8 L glass spinners containing 5 L of culture. They were then turned over to the plant operators for inoculation into fermentors. The plant foreman and operators were responsible for the fermentor system, the cell removal system, and the concentration of antibody in the spent medium via the Pellicon ultrafiltration system. The purification technician was responsible for maintaining and operating the purification systems (protein A column, fraction collector, etc.).

The production plant was operated with a single 8-hr active shift and was monitored during the remaining 16 hr by remote alarms or by regular visits by plant operators from other production areas. The runs were scheduled to exclude weekend activities, with the exception of monitoring the fermentors.

The QA and QC units were comprised of one and three persons, respectively. During production periods these individuals were fully committed to the support of the production unit. The QA officer was responsible for ensuring that methods, equipment, and facilities complied with GMPs and the 9.2.27 Drug Master File. Any deviations from the defined process had to be approved by this individual before the resulting product was allowed to be pooled with previously accepted material. Prior to beginning production the QA unit officer set up a GMP training program and ensured that each individual involved in the effort went through this program. The QC unit was responsible for developing acceptance criteria for raw materials used in the production effort and for applying appropriate tests to these materials prior to their release for use in manufacturing. This group was also responsible for all in-process assays and for chemical tests applied to the final product.

Indirect support was also provided by an individual whose function was performance of the ELISA assay and by the Central Diagnostics Laboratory

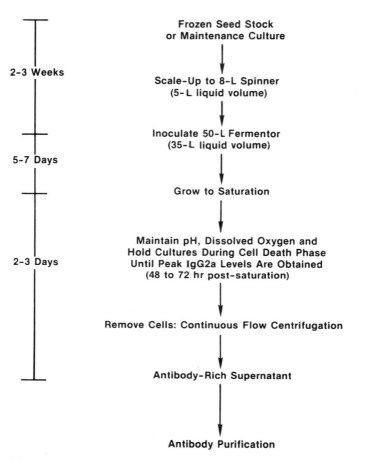

(a)

Figure 4   a. Production process flow: 9.2.27 monoclonal antibody. The time required to progress from a frozen ampule of the 9.2.27 hybridoma to the recovery of antibody-rich supernatant is shown. b. Antibody purification process flow: 9.2.27 monoclonal antibody. The time required for processing the cell-free, antibody-rich supernatant to final bulk product is shown. The figure does not include time required to perform final product testing.

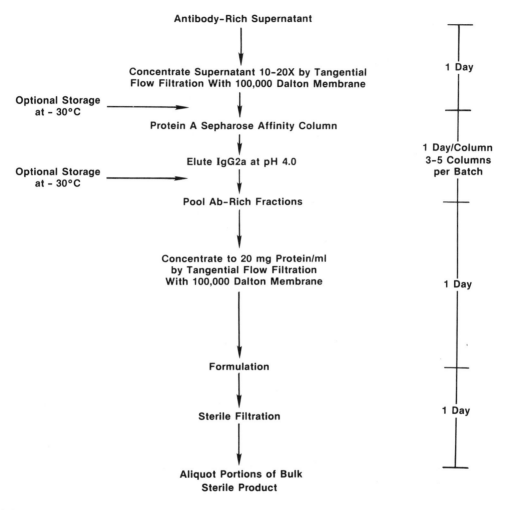

(b)

Figure 4   (Continued)

operated at the NCI-Frederick Cancer Research Facility by Mr. Richard Del Giudice. These laboratories offered endotoxin testing via the limulus amebocyte lysis (LAL) test as well as USP sterility tests and mycoplasma tests performed on seed stocks and final product.

IV. LARGE-SCALE PRODUCTION

Large-scale production actually began prior to true GMP production. Two full-scale production runs were performed using procedures and methods constructed for the GMP campaign to validate that these procedures would, in fact, result in the production of material of acceptable quality. The product of this non-GMP validation effort was designated lot XX03. After evaluating this product and making the appropriate process modifications, GMP production began. The product of this effort, incorporating six production batches, was designated lot F10001.

A. Process Flow

Based on earlier studies referred to above and early studies by Dr. S.-M. Lee and others on methods for purifying the 9.2.27 monoclonal antibody from culture medium (13), a flow chart for large-scale production was developed. The basic outline for this process and an associated time line are shown in Figure 4. Overlapping various phases of the process allowed for production of approximately 280 L of spent medium every 2 weeks.

The cultures were scaled-up from single cryopreserved ampules or ongoing maintenance cultures in 500 ml spinner flasks, according to the scheme shown in Figure 5. The level of serum was reduced from 10% to 8% at the 8 L spinner stage and again to 7% upon inoculation into the fermentor. The 9.2.27 hybridoma was easy to maintain according to this schedule and was extremely predictable in culture. Seed stocks rarely failed to maintain high viabilities and short doubling times (9–15 hr).

Once it was determined that the 8 L spinner cultures fit the limits of acceptability, the fermentors, each containing 30 L of complete medium, were inoculated with 5 L of seed culture. Inoculation was performed through a silicone septum with a specially designed needle. The seed culture was pumped into the fermentor through medical-grade silicone tubing with a peristaltic pump.

Fermentor cultures were grown to saturation. This usually took 4–5 days, during which time the operators maintained pH and dissolved oxygen (DO) at established limits (pH 7.0 ± 0.3; DO > 10% saturation). Both pH and DO were controlled by sparging or overlaying the cultures with air or CO_2. Agitation rates were maintained at approximately 4000 cm/min (tip speed of a .

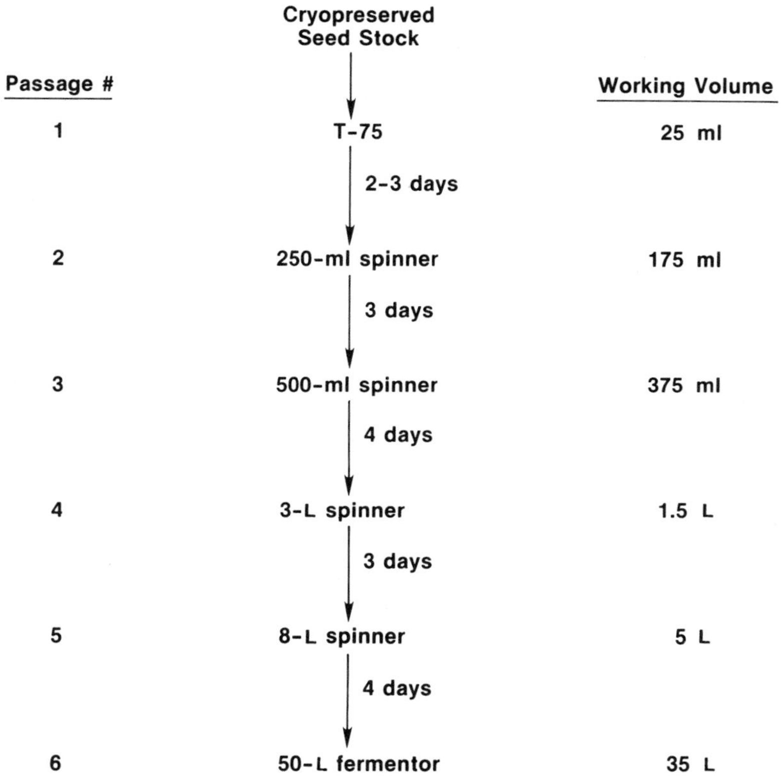

Passage #	Cryopreserved Seed Stock	Working Volume
	↓	
1	T-75	25 ml
	2-3 days	
	↓	
2	250-ml spinner	175 ml
	3 days	
	↓	
3	500-ml spinner	375 ml
	4 days	
	↓	
4	3-L spinner	1.5 L
	3 days	
	↓	
5	8-L spinner	5 L
	4 days	
	↓	
6	50-L fermentor	35 L

Figure 5   Scale-up of 9.2.27 hybridoma: time required to move a frozen ampule of 9.2.27 cells through each stage of expansion up to the 50 L fermentor. Passage number is also shown. Alternatively, cells were held at a maintenance level in the 500 ml spinner until required for a production run, thus shortening the time required for scale-up. Seed stocks were tested for mycoplasma, sterility, viruses (MAP, XC, and S^+/L^- tests), and were submitted for isoenzyme analysis prior to being released by QA for production.

single marine impeller). Once saturation was obtained the cultures were held
at operating parameters through the log death phase of the cultures, which
were chilled when viability reached <20%. A typical growth curve is shown
in Figure 6.

During the fermentor phase of the production samples were taken to
assess antibody production. Figure 7 shows the viability and antibody titer
profiles of three fermentor cultures during a typical production run. After
the cultures were chilled and the terminal antibody titer of each obtained,
the cells were removed by passage through the continuous flow centrifuge
and the cell-free supernatant was held overnight in a chilled stainless steel
holding tank.

The next phase of the operation involved concentration of the antibody
using 100,000 dalton polysulfone membranes in a Pellicon unit. The set-up
for the filtration unit, the operating parameters, and a materials balance from
a typical run are shown in Figure 8. Immediately before and after each use
the assembled unit with accessories (pump, piping, membranes) was cleaned,
sanitized, and depyrogenated with a 52.5 ppm sodium hypochlorite solution.
Contact time was a minimum of 4 hr. The unit was then flushed with
copious amounts of RODI water followed by depyrogenated water. When
rinse water quality equaled the quality of the feed water (in terms of pH,
conductivity, and oxidizable substances) the unit was ready for use. The
unit was deproteinized after each use, immediately prior to cleaning, with a
1M sodium hydroxide solution. The supernatant was pumped with a sanitary
design rotary lobed pump through flexible stainless steel transfer lines to the
Pellicon unit. Antibody was retained by the membranes and was recycled
back into the holding tank while water and molecular species of less than
100,000 daltons passed into the filtrate line, thus reducing the volume of
supernatant and concentrating the antibody. The use of a prewash solution
containing DMEM plus 5% FCS and a postprocessing wash of DMEM alone
provided high recovery rates (>90%).

Antibody was usually concentrated 10-20 times by this method. The
end product, approximately 10-15 L of concentrated 9.2.27 monoclonal
antibody was referred to as *prepurified product* at this stage of the process.
This material was pumped through 2.0 μm positively charged filters (Pall
Trincor Corp., Zeta potential filters) to remove cell debris and loaded as
1.5 L aliquot portions into sterile 2 L roller bottles. This was then stored at
$-30°C$ until it was removed for column purification, usually after 1-2 weeks.

The results of two typical column runs are shown in Table 5. Specific
details of the protein A-Sepharose CL-4B column chromatography purification method are addressed in Chapter 11 and only generally here. This one-
step purification resulted in an approximately 60-120-fold purification of the

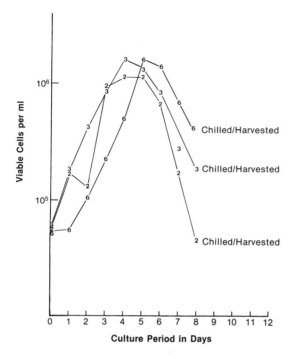

Figure 6 Typical growth of 9.2.27 hybridoma culture in 50-L fermentors: growth curve for production run F06001. Data were collected from fermentors 2, 3, and 6. The short "lag" periods for 2 and 6 are attributed to a short period during which pH went out of range (pH 7.0 ± 0.3).

antibody contained in the prepurified product. Purification levels exceeding 100-fold are likely a reflection of ELISA variability. The purified antibody, now referred to as *purified product*, was again frozen at −30°C in 1-1.5 L aliquot portions in roller bottles. Routine protein assays and ELISA indicated that short-term storage under these conditions did not result in significant changes in product. It should be reemphasized here that all column reagents, washes, buffers, etc., were prepared with depyrogenated water and were made fresh for each column run to control endotoxin levels. A typical production run usually produced sufficient prepurified product for three to five column runs. Loading was usually kept at 2-4 g antibody per column run. During down times or between column runs the column was stored in a 0.02% sodium azide solution. Obviously, use of this preservative required

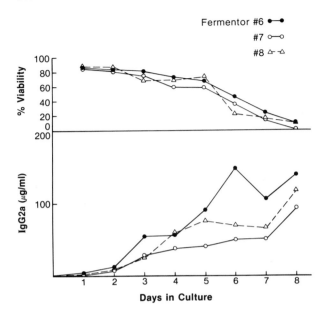

Figure 7 9.2.27 monoclonal antibody production. The antibody titers and viability of three fermentor cultures (6, 7, and 8) are shown. Data were collected during a single production run. Fermentors were harvested on day 8. The reason for the sudden increase and decrease in titer for fermentor 6 between days 5 and 7 is unclear, but it might have been due to assay variability.

extensive washing of the column with validation by QC that all azide was removed prior to reuse.

B. Final Product

When sufficient quantities of purified antibody had been prepared from several production runs, these "sublots" were removed from frozen storage for final concentration and formulation to final bulk product form. The concentration was performed with the Pellicon unit fitted with 15 ft² of 100,000 dalton polysulfone membranes. Starting titers in the purified product pool averaged 1 mg/ml. The antibody was concentrated to 25 mg/ml using a peristaltic pump to drive the material across the Pellicon membranes at a feed pressure of 10–15 psig and a back-pressure of ~5 psig. After the proper concentration was achieved, the feed line to the Pellicon was

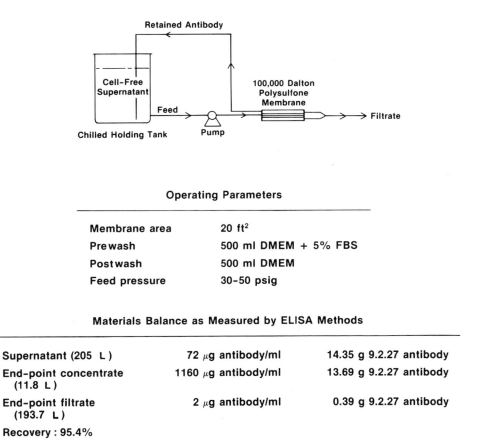

Figure 8 Concentration of 9.2.27 monoclonal antibody in cell-free supernatant: physical set-up of the tangential flow ultrafiltration system. Also shown are the operating parameters and the materials balance from a typical production run. Using the pre- and postwashes consistently provided recovery rates of >90%. It is assumed that the prewash (with serum) helped reduce nonspecific adsorption of the antibody to the membranes and that the postwash with DMEM alone helped remove gel-polarized antibody from the membrane surface.

Table 5 Purification of 9.2.27 Monoclonal Antibody by Protein A-Sepharose Column Chromatography[a]

Process stage	Total antibody (g)		Total protein (g)		Specific activity (mg antibody/ mg protein)		Purification[b] (fold)		Yield[c] (%)	
	Run 1	Run 4	Run 1	Run 4	Run 1	Run 4	Run 1	Run 4	Run 1	Run 4
Prepurified product[d]	2.5	5.5	101	275	0.024	0.020	—	—	—	—
Purified product[e]	2.8	3.7	1.0	2.2	2.9	1.6	120	82	110	67

[a]Data collected from two typical production runs. Operational parameters are described in the text.
[b]Purification (fold): Specific activity of purified product ÷ specific activity of prepurified product.
[c]Yield: (Total antibody in purified product ÷ Total antibody in prepurified product) × 100.
[d]Prepurified product is antibody-rich concentrate obtained after 10–20× concentration of cell-free supernatant by 100,000 dalton cut-off ultrafiltration but before affinity purification.
[e]Purified product is antibody-rich fractions eluted from the affinity column.
Data kindly provided by Dr. Shwu-Maan Lee, Program Resources, Inc., NCI-FCRF.

Table 6   Biological and Chemical Analysis[a] of 9.2.27 Monoclonal Antibody Final Bulk Product

Assay	Results	
	Lot XX03	Lot F10001
Mouse IgG (mg/ml)	19.0	19.2
Endotoxin (ng/ml)[b]	15.1	17.5
Protein A (ng/ml)	72.0	3.9
Bovine IgG (mg/ml)	1.05	0.38
USP sterility tests	Negative	Negative
Mycoplasma test	Negative	Negative
Reverse transcriptase activity	Negative	Negative
Specific activity (mg antibody/ mg protein)	0.98	1.2
DNA (μg/ml)	2.62[c]	Not available[d]
Potassium (mg/ml)	3.5	3.2
Sodium (mg/ml)	10.5	9.5
Chloride (mg/ml)	17.2	16.7
Orthophosphate (mg/ml)	4.4	5.1
pH	6.8	6.7
Protein (mg/ml)	19.3	15.6
HPLC	<1% impurities	<1% impurities
SDS-PAGE	<10% impurities	<10% impurities
Isoelectric point[e]	7.5, 7.3, 7.1, 6.9, 6.8, 6.7, and 6.6	7.5, 7.3, 7.1, 6.9, 6.8, and 6.7

[a]Data kindly provided by Dr. Shwu-Maan Lee, Program Resources, Inc., NCI-FCRF.
[b]As determined by Limulus amebocyte lysis assay.
[c]Fluorescence assay. Discontinued after lot XX03 due to limited sensitivity.
[d]Hybridization assay was attempted but results were unclear, presumably due to interference by large amounts of protein. Further analysis was not performed in this facility on this bulk product.
[e]This charge heterogeneity may be related to variations in glycosylation and in posttranslational modifications (17).

disconnected from the antibody reservoir and reconnected to a flask containing a measured amount of sterile buffer. This was used to sweep the membranes and lines of the Pellicon and was then directed back into the antibody reservoir. In this manner some of the antibody that had formed a gel-polarized layer on the membranes was recovered and the final bulk material was simultaneously diluted to approximately 20 mg/ml.

Formulation was achieved by additions of sodium chloride until the proper chloride level was obtained. Following QC analysis and validation that desired parameters (pH, purity measured by HPLC and SDS-PAGE, chemical identity tests, etc.) had been obtained the bulk material was passed through a 0.22 μm sterile filter and into sterile glass serum bottles. This material was then referred to as *final bulk product*.

Two lots of 9.2.27 monoclonal antibody were prepared in a 5-month period using the methods described in this chapter. The first lot, XX03, required two production runs. Approximately six production runs were required to produce lot F10001. The final product analyses of these lots are shown in Table 6. The total yield of final bulk product from this system was 11 g antibody in lot XX03 and 32 g antibody in lot F10001. These values are based upon ELISA determinations.

V. CONCLUSIONS

While it is possible to develop a system, albeit a simple one, for obtaining large quantities of a monoclonal antibody from conventional fermentors and by the use of a one-step affinity chromatography purification system, some points should be stressed.

A. Expense

We found this system to be fairly expensive. Estimated costs were approximately $5000/g of finished bulk product. A large portion of this cost was for start-up (facility modifications, capital equipment) and for time required for development of the QA/QC package for GMP compliance (procedures, worksheets, validation of processes and equipment, environmental monitoring, construction of the 9.2.27, Drug Master File, etc.). Subsequent production efforts, however, can draw upon these resources thus reducing considerably the cost per gram.

B. Impact of GMPs

The transition of a facility such as this one from conventional research and development to regulated production of a biological under GMPs was not simple. Participants had to develop an understanding of the role of QA and QC. Front-line personnel needed to understand the reasons for instructional worksheets and written procedures for operations they might have performed hundreds of times previously. It was important for operators to have ready access at all times to the documentation provided by QA for manufacturing the antibody. Deviations from any procedure had to be recorded, reviewed, discussed, and, finally, accepted by the QA officer prior to acceptance of a lot of product.

The benefit of the GMP program became obvious once the campaign was constructed and on-line. Decision-making became more "by the book," thus taking some of the stress off of front-line personnel who previously may have felt compelled to make quick "off-the-cuff" decisions.

C. Problems

The production methods described here were fairly simple to manage and maintain. Minor problems with an occasionally contaminated fermentor or one that failed to grow to an acceptable density or to produce sufficient product were easy to deal with: the affected culture was simply excluded from further processing. These incidences were rare even though no antibiotics were used in scale-up or production medium. Problems related to final product composition are addressed in general below and in greater detail in Dr. S.-M. Lee's chapter (Chap. 11) and journal article (15).

A subtle problem we were not able to fully resolve was the presence of residual endotoxin in the final bulk product. We had not developed, at that time, a reliable method for reducing the endotoxin level in a product like the 9.2.27 monoclonal antibody. Our approach to this was to screen all raw materials used in the process; to use fresh, depyrogenated water (≤ 0.014 ng/ml endotoxin) for all product-contact buffers and equipment rinses; to perform routine sampling of all product-containing materials throughout the production run; and to exclude sublots of purified product with high endotoxin levels in the preparation of final bulk product. With these methods, endotoxin levels through column elution (purified product) but before final ultrafiltration concentration were kept to approximately 1.0 ng/ml.

It was expected that final concentration of product with 100,000 dalton polysulfone membranes would not concentrate endotoxin ($<100,000$ daltons) along with the antibody but might actually assist in reducing the level. However, in preparing both lots of antibody we found that endotoxin was concentrated almost but not quite linearly with the antibody. It is assumed that this was due to the formation of micelles or aggregates of endotoxin resulting in a molecular size larger than 100,000 daltons and also due to some "apparent" reduction in membrane porosity due to the formation of a gel-polarized layer of antibody on the membrane surface. The formation of this layer was controllable to a degree by careful control of the ultrafiltration process. However, as the antibody concentration increased to the desired level of 25 mg/ml, it became impossible to control polarization with the physical means available (sweeping the membrane, flushing the system with buffer, backpulsing the membrane with buffer). By careful application of these techniques, however, we were able to recover up to 9 g antibody from this polarized layer.

Once the level of endotoxin in the final product, prior to sterile filling of product bottles, was ascertained and found to be greater than 10 ng/ml several methods were attempted to reduce it. Two of these were: (a) use of charge-modified filters (Pall Trincor Corp., Posidyne 2 μm filter) and (b) adsorption of endotoxin with aluminum oxide gel or Detoxi-gel (Pierce). The first method removed small amounts of endotoxin as well as nearly equal amounts of antibody. The second method resulted in complete loss of endotoxin and antibody (aluminum oxide gel) or no loss of endotoxin (Detoxi-gel) (15).

Use of protein A-Sepharose CL-4B, while efficient for rapid recovery of the antibody, resulted in low levels of protein A contamination (see Table 6). The same column was used for lots XX03 and F10001. The decrease in protein A in the second lot (F10001) of antibody is likely due to the fact that most of the protein A capable of being leached from the column was removed in the early column runs (lot XX03). This has recently been reported in literature by Dertzbaugh et al. (16).

The presence of bovine IgG in the final product is likely due to the use of fetal calf serum in the production medium and subsequent copurification of some of this material.

The presence of residual amounts of DNA in the first lot of material may be the result of cell death, which could be attributable to process design (holding cultures until <20% viability, shear forces exterted by centrifugation, etc.). Results for the second lot were not obtained due to difficulties experienced with the hybridization assay in the presence of large amounts of protein.

Although some of these problems might preclude clinical use of the final product in its bulk form, the use of large-scale fermentor cultures was shown to be a reliable method for producing gram quantities of monoclonal antibody. Use of serum-free or reduced serum medium, process modifications to limit shear, stringent control of raw materials to keep endotoxin at a low level, and extensive prewashing of the affinity column to remove leachable protein A, may result in a reasonable process for producing bulk material suitable for clinical use. Reliable, efficient methods for removal of endotoxin from such products prior to sterile filling would most certainly improve the usefulness of this system.

ACKNOWLEDGMENTS

I would like to extend my thanks to the following people who supported this project: Dr. M. C. Flickinger, Dr. S.-M. Lee, Dr. G. Muschik, Dr. M. Gustafson, Dr. R. Herberman, Dr. A. C. Morgan, Jr., Ivan Lufriu, Irving Jones, Dana Pickle, Pam Clark, Chuck Collins, Dave Herber, Chris Clabaugh, Robert Ricketts, Penny Hylton, Marie Wroble, Mark Dertzbaugh, Frederick Klein, Judy Holian, Ralph Hopkins III, Lorraine Beall, and Keith Nuttle.

This research was sponsored, at least in part, by the National Cancer Institute, DHHS, under contract NO1-CO-23910 with Program Resources, Incorporated. The contents of this publication do not necessarily reflect the views or policies of the DHHS, nor does mention of trade names, commercial products, or organizations imply endorsement by the U.S. Government.

REFERENCES

1. Kohler, G. and Milstein, C. (1975). Continuous cultures of fused cells secreting antibody of predetermined specificity. *Nature 256*: 495–497.
2. Kohler, G. and Milstein, C. (1976). Derivation of specific antibody producing tissue culture and tumor lines by cell fusion. *Eur. J. Immunol. 6*: 511–519.
3. Lebherz, W. B. III, Lee, S.-M., Gustafson, M. E., Ricketts, R. T., Lufriu, I. F., Morgan, A. C., and Flickinger, M. C. (1985). Production of monoclonal antibody by large-scale submerged hybridoma cultures. *In Vitro 21*: 16A.
4. Dillman, R. O. and Royston, I. (1984). Applications of monoclonal antibodies in cancer therapy. *Br. Med. Bull. 40*: 240–246.
5. Hofstaetter, T., Gronski, P., and Seiler, F. R. (1984). Immunotoxins—theoretical and practical aspects. *Behring Inst. Mitt. 74*: 113–121.
6. Blair, A. H. and Glose, T. I. (1983). Linkage of cytotoxic agents to immunoglobulins. *J. Immunol. Methods 59*: 129–143.
7. Oldham, R. K. (1983). Monoclonal antibodies in cancer therapy. *J. Clin. Oncol. 1*: 582–590.
8. Cleveland, W. L., Wood, I., and Erlanger, B. F. (1983). Routine large-scale production of monoclonal antibodies in a protein-free culture medium. *J. Immunol. Methods 56*: 221–234.
9. Morgan, A. C. Jr., Galloway, D. R., and Reisfeld, R. A. (1981). Production and characterization of monoclonal antibody to a melanoma specific glycoprotein. *Hybridoma 1*: 27–36.
10. Morgan, A. C. Jr. (1982). Monoclonal antibodies to human melanoma-associated antigens. In *Elicitation and Evaluation With Immunochemically*

Defined Antigen Preparations in Melanoma Antigens and Antibodies. Edited by R. A. Reisfeld and S. Ferrone. New York, Plenum Publishing, pp. 279–288.

11. Zwerner, R. K., Cox, R. M., Lynn, J. D., and Acton, R. T. (1981). Five year perspective of the large-scale growth of mammalian cells in suspension culture. *Biotech. Bioeng. 23*: 2717–2735.

12. Feder, J. and Tolbert, W. R. (1983). The large-scale cultivation of mammalian cells. *Sci. Am. 248*: 36–43.

13. de St. Groth, S. F. (1983). Automated production of monoclonal antibodies in a cryostat. *J. Immunol. Methods 57*: 121–136.

14. Abrams, P. G., Ochs, J. J., Giardina, S. L., Morgan, A. C., Wilburn, S. B., Wilt, A. R., Oldham, R. K., and Foon, K. A. (1984). Production of large quantities of human immunoglobulin in the ascites of athymic mice: Implications for the development of anti-human idiotype monoclonal antibodies. *J. Immunol. 132*: 1611–1613.

15. Lee, S.-M., Gustafson, M. E., Pickle, D. J., Flickinger, M. C., Muschik, G. M., and Morgan, A. C. Jr. (1986). Large-scale purification of a murine antimelanoma monoclonal antibody. *J. Biotech. 4*: 189–204.

16. Dertzbaugh, M. T., Flickinger, M. C., and Lebherz, W. B. III. (1985). An enzyme immunoassay for the detection of Staphylococcal protein A in affinity-purified products. *J. Immunol. Methods 83*: 169–177.

17. Staines, N. A. (1983). Monoclonal antibodies. In *Biochemical Research Techniques.* Edited by J. M. Wrigglesworth. New York, John Wiley, pp. 177–209.

7

Monoclonal Antibody Production in a Ceramic Matrix

JAMES E. PUTNAM
Lilly Research Laboratories, A Division of Eli Lilly and Company, Indianapolis, Indiana

I. INTRODUCTION

Production of large amounts of monoclonal antibody is becoming increasingly important as new uses are being found (1). Several methods are currently being used for large scale in vitro culture of hybridomas. Homogeneous suspension cultures such as those used in fermentation of bacteria have been successful in many cases (2), but this type culture method has disadvantages. Some cells are sensitive to the shear forces seen during the culture agitation and the separation of product from the culture can be difficult. Other methods that address these problems include encapsulation of the cells in a semipermeable membrane (3), or immobilization of the culture in packed beds (4), on membranes (5), or within hollow fibers (4,6,7), but these may cause other problems in large-scale applications.

Described here is a system based on the immobilization of the hybridoma culture on a ceramic matrix coupled with the ability to maintain and control the culture parameters (8-10). The ability to maintain and control culture pH and oxygen levels has been shown to be very important in the overall productivity of a culture (4,11).

Immobilization of the cells can have many advantages in hybridoma culture. An immobilized culture produces waste products at one-quarter to one-half the rate observed with actively growing cells (12). The product can be harvested without removal of a corresponding number of cells either in a batch process or in continuous feed and harvest mode. In addition, the culture does not need to divide constantly, which may allow for increased productivity.

II. OPTICELL SYSTEM

The OPTICELL Culture System, shown in Figure 1, is an automated system designed for the large scale production of animal cells, both attachment-dependent and attachment-independent. The system's versatility results from the use of two types of ceramic matrices used as growth chambers. One allows for the attachment and growth of attachment-dependent cells with the ability for complete harvest of the culture using conventional methods. The second ceramic allows for the immobilization of non-attachment-dependent cells, such as hybridoma cells, but complete cell harvest becomes difficult. The ceramic matrices are rigid structures that provide a large surface area for immobilization in a relatively small volume. The matrix, as shown in Figure 2, is cylindrical with many small square channels running throughout the length of the core. The dimensions of the matrix are approximately 30.6 cm in length and 9.1 cm in diameter, with a channel size of approximately 1.2 mm^2. The ceramic matrix is encapsulated in a set of plastic endcaps, which allow medium to flow through the matrix. To ensure even flow through the square channels, flow diverters are incorporated into the endcaps at the inlet and outlet sides. The entire matrix is incorporated into a flow loop, and medium is perfused continuously through the core and over the immobilized culture.

Figure 3 shows the schematic of the flow path in the bioreactor cabinet. The oxygen content and pH of the medium are monitored continuously by autoclavable probes in two probe chambers, both before and after the medium is perfused through the growth chamber. Information from these probes is relayed to the integrated controller, which compares the actual values to setpoints the operator has entered into a computer. The oxygen-in (O_2 in) probe controls the amount of oxygen gas that flows through the inline gas permeators, so that the oxygen content of the medium entering the culture is at a constant value. The oxygen-out (O_2 out) probe controls the speed of the main pump. When the O_2-out value drops below the setpoint, the pump speed will automatically increase and pass more medium and more oxygen over the culture, thus raising the O_2-out reading. The pH-in (pH in) probe determines the flow of carbon dioxide through the permeators, as well as controlling the auxiliary pump, which adds sodium bicarbonate or sodium hydroxide to the medium. These controlling features help maintain the

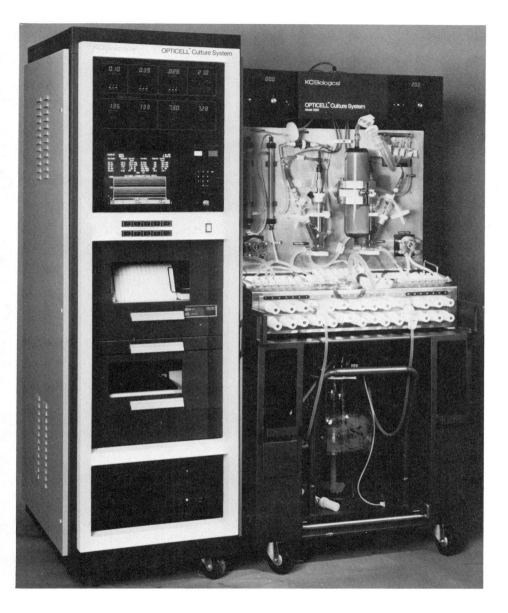

Figure 1 OPTICELL Culture System. On the left is the integrated controller, to the right is the bioreactor cabinet containing the ceramic matrix. The matrix is located on the center of the stainless steel shelf, in the vertical position.

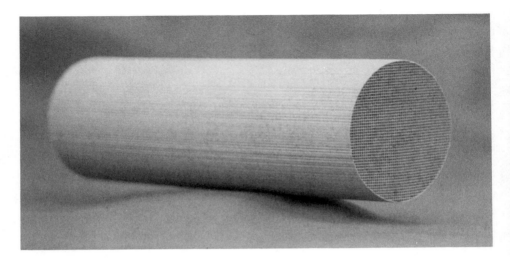

Figure 2 Photo of the ceramic matrix that provides for immobilization of non-attachment-dependent cells. It is 9.1 cm in diameter, 30.6 cm in length, with a channel size of approximately 1.2 mm^2.

oxygen content and pH of the medium at constant values throughout the run. By altering the setpoints, the absolute oxygen and pH levels can be changed, to aid in determining the best values for optimal productivity.

The integrated controller, in addition to controlling gas flow and pump speed, stores all the information and provides a printout with the culture parameters, such as pH, pump speed, etc. Since the culture is immobilized, the computer can calculate the oxygen consumption rate (OCR) of the culture. This is done by subtracting the oxygen content of the medium after it flows over the culture from the oxygen content of the medium before it passes over the culture, then multiplying by a constant to convert the amount of dissolved oxygen to μmoles, after taking into account the flow rate of the medium through the growth chamber. The OCR has been shown to parallel the growth curve of a culture, as well as indicate overall culture respiration. The OCR is included in the printout, and provision is made for entering the product concentrations. It or any other parameter can be displayed graphically at any time. This information, especially the OCR, is very useful in optimizing culture productivity (see below).

The integrated controller also provides a backup power supply so that if the power should be interrupted, the computer will continue to run and store data. Should the gas supply run out, the controller will automatically

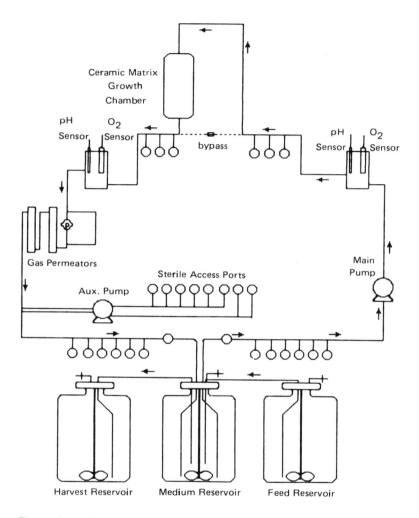

Figure 3 Schematic of the OPTICELL System, incorporating the ceramic matrix. Medium is recirculated through the loop, as indicated by the arrows, with peristaltic pumps (Cole Parmer) utilizing silicon tubing. Oxygen levels and pH are monitored by autoclavable probes from Instrumentation Laboratories and Ingold, respectively. The gas permeators consist of glass cylinders containing a bundle of gas permeable silicon tubing potted at each end. A controlled mixture of N_2, O_2, and CO_2 gas is passed through the lumen at pressures of 1–4 psi. The medium flows around the exterior of the bundle, gas exchange across the silicon tubing takes place by diffusion. The harvest reservoir and feed reservoir are added for continuous feed and harvest; with batch feeding, the entire medium reservoir containing spent medium is replaced with one containing fresh medium.

turn on an air pump to have air flow through the permeators so that the culture will not be lost, although control of oxygen levels and pH may not be possible.

Access to the main flow loop for such operations as cell seeding, bicarbonate addition, product removal, addition of growth factors, or other uses is provided for by sterile connect/disconnect ports incorporated into the loop. These several ports are intended to be used only once per run, so that the sterility of the system will not be compromised. The entire flow loop and the stainless steel shelf, onto which the loop is incorporated, are autoclavable for ease of sterilization. A presterilized ceramic growth chamber is connected to the loop using quick connect/disconnects.

The bioreactor cabinet can be used in a warm room or rolled into a standard roller bottle cabinet for regulation of temperature. A portable laminar flow hood is available so that all connections can be made in a HEPA-filtered, clean air environment, without the need to roll the cabinet into a downflow or clean room. The integrated controller can be put in the warm room or left outside. If the unit is being used in a restricted-access location, a remote monitor can be added so that the culture can be monitored from a central or safe area.

To inoculate and maintain the attachment-independent cells on the ceramic with the OPTICELL Culture System, the following protocols are used. To initiate cell inoculation, the system is filled with 20–40 L medium and a small vessel is added to quick connect/disconnects so that the vessel, ceramic, and the auxiliary pump form a small loop. The vessel is filled with 100 ml medium and 33% of the cell inoculum of 10^9 cells is added. The medium is then recirculated for 10 min at 750 ml/min with the ceramic in a vertical position. This gives an even distribution of cells throughout the core. After the recirculation, the core is turned to a horizontal position so that one of the four sides of the square channels is flat, allowing the cells to fall onto the surface. After a settling period of 15 min, the core is put in a vertical position and 22% of the cell inoculum is added to the vessel, followed by a recirculation period of 5 min at 750 ml/min. The ceramic is turned to a horizontal position and the cells allowed to settle for 15 min on the second side of the square channels. This cycle of recirculation and settling is repeated until all four sides are seeded. After this, the ceramic is allowed to sit with no flow for 1 hr to let the cells condition the medium. Then flow is started through the entire system flow loop including the ceramic matrix with the matrix held in a horizontal position throughout the run. Flow rates throughout the run are varied from 0.16 to 1.0 L/min total flow, and are dependent on the oxygen usage of the culture.

III. IMMOBILIZATION OF CELLS

Table 1 summarizes some of the immobilization data from various hybridomas grown in the OPTICELL System. The percentage immobilized cells on day 0 was determined by counting the number of cells in suspension in the system after the ceramic was seeded with 10^9 cells. The percentage of 20-8-4S cells (American Type Culture Collection HB-11) immobilized on day 3 was determined by counting the cells in suspension in the system, and comparing this to the number of cells immobilized in the system. The number of immobilized cells was determined by counting the number of cells that can be removed from the ceramic by increasing the flow through the core to 12 L/min, and then adding the number of cells left immobilized on the core. This number was determined by assaying the amount of DNA left on the core after the harvest procedure. The total cells immobilized in the system using the standard-size core ranged between 3 and 10×10^{10} cells, depending on the cell line and the day of harvest.

The cells that are not immobilized on the core are simply recirculated through the system. Cell traps can be incorporated into the flow loop to remove these circulating cells, but this has not been found to be necessary, since the number of cells in suspension has been quite low. When the ceramic matrix is left in a horizontal position, it appears that many of the recirculating cells are reattaching on subsequent passes through the core, to be replaced by other cells released from the core. Overall, the number of cells in suspension during a run remains constant, with 70-95% of the recirculating cells viable.

The surface of the matrix used for suspension cells is rough to the touch and quite porous. Microscopically, as shown in Figure 4, the ceramic surface can be seen to have many small, irregular pores that travel throughout the walls, much like a sponge. During the seeding procedure, the cells have an opportunity to settle along the wall and fall into the holes or crevices. The topography of the ceramic surface coupled with the characteristic laminar flow of medium through the channels protects the cells from shear forces that could cause dislodgement. As these entrapped cells divide, they then become tightly packed in the matrix, providing a very effective means of immobilization. Cells that tend to form clumps in suspension or that will loosely attach to a surface are better able to remain immobilized in the ceramic. However, even cells that do not show a tendency to attach to a surface show a high percentage of immobilization, which tends to increase over time.

The OPTICELL Culture System has been used on a wide variety of hybridomas, with both mouse and human parents. In all cases the cells were immobilized and able to be cultured for long time periods; many runs lasted several months.

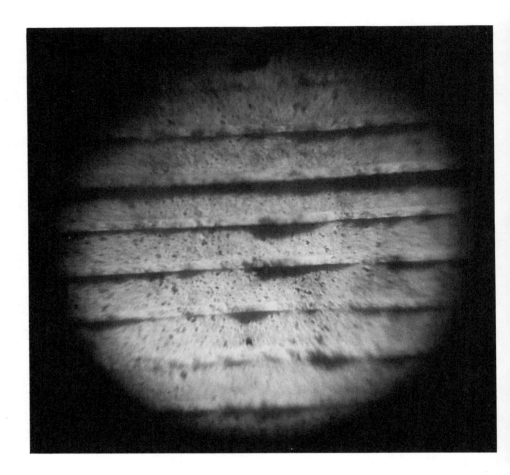

Figure 4   Magnified view of the porous ceramic surface used for immobilization of attachment-independent cells shows holes that travel throughout the wall and provide for cell immobilization.

Table 1 Cell Immobilization on the Ceramic Matrix

Cell	Type	Antibody produced	Cell characteristics in flasks	% Immobilization		
				Day 0	Day 3	Day 14
SP2/0	Mouse	–	Single cells	85	–	–
20-8-4S[a]	Mouse-mouse	IgG	Single cells	>99	80	90
7D7G9[b]	Human-human	IgM	Clumps	>99	>99	98
80-13.6[c]	Human-mouse	IgM	Loosely attached	>99	99	99
HMB 109	Human-mouse	IgM	Clumps	>99	>99	99

[a]SP2/0 Parent cell line.
[b]UC729-6 Parent cell line.
[c]NS-1 Parent cell line.

IV. BATCH FEEDING VERSUS CONTINUOUS FEED
AND HARVEST

Immobilization of the culture in a perfusion system allows for easier changing of the culture medium. The medium containing the product can easily be removed from the system without disturbing the culture itself. In this way, growth of the culture becomes less important since it is not necessary to replace cells removed during product recovery.

Two major strategies can be used to change the medium in a perfusion system. One can do a batch change, in which the entire medium volume is removed and replaced at once. Alternatively, one can use continuous feed and harvest, in which a small volume of medium is constantly removed and replaced with fresh medium. The overall medium exchange rate is similar to a batch exchange. Both of these strategies have been evaluated in an OPTICELL System. When seeded with 20-8-4S cells, the continuous feed and harvest method gives the best results.

Figure 5 compares the IgG concentration and the oxygen consumption rates of 20-8-4S cells during culture in the OPTICELL in serum-free medium using either batch feeding or continuous feed and harvest. In this experiment, cells were inoculated into the OPTICELL at 10^9 total cells and cultured for 3 days in 40 L RPMI 1640 + 10% fetal bovine serum (FBS). Following this, the medium was batch changed in both systems with 20 L KC 2000, a serum-free medium containing 250 μg/ml total protein (KC Biological), for an additional 2 days. Subsequently, the cells were either maintained with 20-40 L batches of KC 2000 changed every 2-4 days, with an average consumption of 10 L/day, or continuous feed and harvest of KC 2000 at an average exchange rate of 10-12 L/day. At 840 hr (35 days) in the continuous feed and harvest system, the medium was changed to an experimental low-protein medium containing 60 μg/ml total protein. In an effort to concentrate the amount of antibody in the medium seen using the batch medium exchange, at 460 hr (19 days) 40 L medium was left in the system 6 days for an average exchange rate of 7 L/day. Starting at 600 hr (25 days) 20 L were left in the system 6 days, for an average exchange rate of 3 L/day.

IgG concentration in the batch method of medium exchange (40 L replaced every 4 days) started at near zero as fresh medium was added and increased to approximately 35-40 μg/ml after 4 days. When the medium was left in longer, the concentration reached 55 μg/ml, but this was done at the cost of apparent productivity of the culture. Subsequent medium exchanges resulted in very low IgG concentrations, even at the original exchange rate of 10 L/day, although the cells were using oxygen and were apparently alive. This is strong evidence that the cells must be supplied with sufficient medium at all times. Once they are starved for medium, production falls rapidly and does not quickly return.

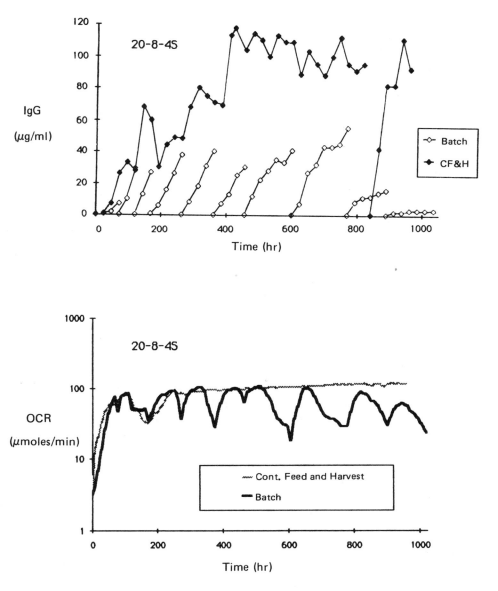

Figure 5 IgG concentration and OCR of the 20-8-4S cell line grown in serum-free medium using either batch feeding or continuous feed and harvest. Medium consumption was approximately 10–12 L/day in both cases, except at 450–750 hr in batch feeding, where the medium supplied was reduced in an effort to increase IgG concentration (see text).

Continuous feed and harvest of the medium at an average exchange rate of 10-12 L/day resulted in the IgG concentrations climbing to approximately 100 μg/ml after 17 days and remaining at that level for over 3 weeks. When the medium was batch exchanged with the experimental medium containing 60 μg/ml total protein at 840 hr, followed by continuous feed and harvest, IgG production again went to near 100 μg/ml, or over g/day amounts.

The OCR of the culture in a batch medium exchange exhibited a repeating pattern. First the OCR rose when fresh medium was added, then it remained steady for several hours, after which it decreased as the medium became depleted or waste products accumulated. The cycle repeated with each new addition of fresh medium. With continuous feed and harvest, a high OCR was maintained for long periods without the large fluctuations seen in the batch feeding, even though the rate of medium usage was the same in both methods. This constant or slowly rising OCR implies that the culture is being maintained in a constant and healthy condition, apparently providing for the higher antibody concentration and production.

Cumulative IgG produced by the two methods varied considerably (Fig. 6). In 40 days using the batch method of exchange, 8.7 g IgG was produced; using continuous feed and harvest, 38 g was produced during the same time period. This was an increase of >330% with only a slight increase in medium consumption.

When the 20-8-4S cell line was cultured using traditional methods, it produced a maximum concentration of 20-30 μg/ml IgG in flasks and 25-35 μg/ml in spinner cultures, using either KC 2000 or medium containing 1% FBS, over 4 days. A partial medium exchange at the rate of 20% per day in the spinner cultures resulted in slightly increased production, 40 μg/ml IgG, using either KC 2000 or medium containing 1% FBS. The increase in productivity seen with the OPTICELL over conventional methods has been reproduced with almost every cell tested. The increase underlines the benefits of using an immobilized cell culture: better maintenance and selection of critical culture parameters.

Determination of the optimal feed rate to be used in continuous feed and harvest is important in producing the maximum amount of product using the least medium without compromising the culture. Several approaches can be used to determine this rate. In the above group of experiments, the feed rate was determined by analysis of the OCR curve from batch feeding. Using this cell line, 40 L medium would give a rise, plateau, and fall in the OCR over 4 days. This worked out to consumption at 10 L/day, so continuous feed and harvest was set up using approximately this value. If a much greater feed rate is used, we have seen that the culture does not produce additional product, and the amount of antibody/ml is diluted out by the greater

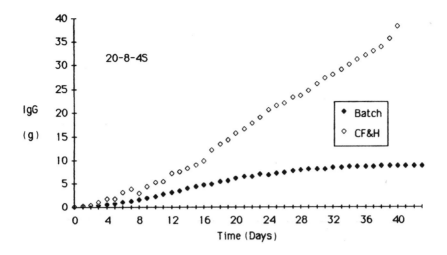

Figure 6   Cumulative IgG produced in the OPTICELL using serum-free medium with batch feeding or continuous feed and harvest methods.

medium volume. The pH of the culture is kept higher, however, due to the addition of more bicarbonate and the dilution of the lactic acid produced by the culture. A much slower feed rate results in a decline in both the OCR and the antibody production.

Another method of determining the continuous feed and harvest rate would be to start continuous feed and harvest at relatively high rate, then slowly decrease the rate until the OCR starts to decline, then increase it back to maintain a steady OCR. However, one of the best ways to determine the feed rate is to monitor a component consumed from the medium, such as glucose. We have found that in general, maintaining the glucose concentration, as determined with a glucose analyzer (Beckman Instruments), at a constant concentration results in the best antibody production with the least medium consumption. A declining glucose concentration suggests the possibility that depletion of other major components may be taking place.

Continuous feed and harvest allows the opportunity to maintain a chemostat-like culture condition. Figure 7 shows the OCR and glucose concentration of two runs. The top graph shows the 20-8-4S line with batch feeding; the bottom half shows the 7D7G9 line with intermittent feeding until 230 hr, at which time continuous feed and harvest was initiated. As indicated, in batch feeding the glucose concentration would fall until there was a medium change, at which time it would jump to a high level and again start to fall.

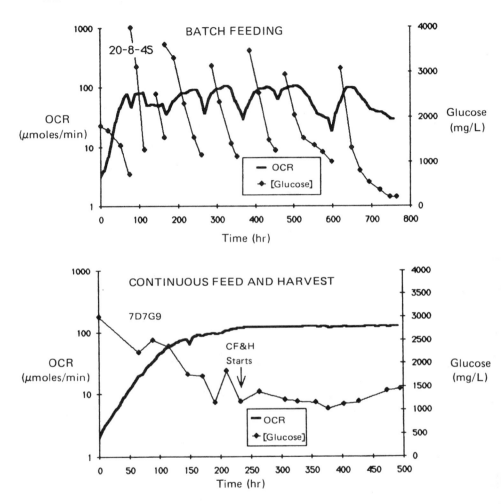

Figure 7 OCR and glucose concentration measured during batch feeding (top) or continuous feed and harvest (bottom). Continuous feed and harvest allows culture nutrients to be maintained at constant levels, and functions as a chemostat.

Using continuous feed and harvest, however, the glucose concentrations remained constant, thus providing similar medium conditions throughout a run. This allowed the cells to adapt readily to a particular environment, and allowed the cells to produce steadily and effectively.

It can be concluded from the above that medium and culture management are very important to the overall productivity of a culture. It is important that a culture be supplied an adequate amount of medium, or else productivity will decline and perhaps not return. It is also apparent that maintaining the culture respiration at a constant state by medium management can have a profound effect on the productivity. This can be done relatively easily by using continuous feed and harvest, especially in an immobilized culture system where constant regrowth of the culture is not necessary.

V. ADDITIONAL BENEFITS OF IMMOBILIZATION, CONTINUOUS FEED AND HARVEST, AND OCR

Using the OCR and continuous feed and harvest allows for benefits in addition to increased culture productivity. The OCR can also be used as an indication of the antibody production rate of a culture.

Figure 8 shows the OCR and antibody production rate from the batch feeding experiment described above. The antibody production was calculated by determining the daily concentration of IgG in the medium using an ELISA assay, calculating the total amount in the entire system, and subtracting the amount that was in the system the previous day. This gives us the amount of IgG produced during each 24 hr period. These points were then plotted at the center of each time frame. The graph indicates that during the first 450 hr of culture there was a high correlation between the OCR and the antibody production rate. Maximum antibody production occurs during peak OCR, indicating that maintenance of the OCR at the maximum level would be productive. After 450 hr the correlation declines. This was apparently due to the medium management used in an effort to increase antibody production. As described previously, when the medium was left in the system for longer and longer periods, the concentration of antibody increased for a short while, but overall productivity declined and fell to near zero. But during the period of healthy maintenance, it was seen that the greatest antibody production was during greatest oxygen consumption. Small changes in culture condition, temperature, etc., have an almost immediate effect on the OCR, and potentially on the antibody production rate. Since the OCR is constantly monitored, one can immediately see the effect the change will have on culture productivity. This information can be very valuable when one is attempting to maximize production. It allows for the instantaneous monitoring of culture productivity without the need to await assay results, sampling, etc.

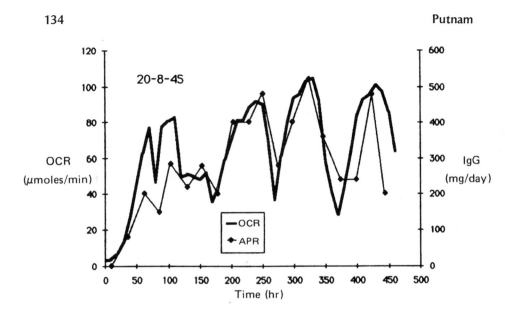

Figure 8 Correlation between OCR and antibody production rate (APR). Hybridoma culture 20-8-4S was maintained in the OPTICELL by batch feeding. Maximum antibody production occurs during peak OCR, indicating that maintenance of OCR at the maximum level would be productive.

Many production protocols call for growing a culture up to high density using a growth medium, then removing the medium and changing it to a maintenance or production medium. Although this change can sometimes be made using a batch change, often the culture must be weaned over to the maintenance medium slowly. Using continuous feed and harvest, it is very easy to wean cells gradually from one type of medium to another, without stressing the culture. Figure 9 shows the OCR curves for three experiments. The 20-8-4S cell line was initiated in 40 L RPMI 1640 with 10% FBS, followed by a complete batch change to serum-free medium at 120 hr. Continuous feed and harvest was started immediately after the batch change of medium. The OCR of the culture decreased over the next 70 hr due to the rapid switch to serum-free medium. After a period of adaptation, the OCR again started to rise, until a fairly steady OCR was reached. The 7D7G9 cell line and the 80-13.6 line (13), a human–human and human–mouse hybridoma, respectively, both producing IgM were initiated in a modified Iscoves medium containing 10% FBS. The 7D7G9 had continuous feed of serum-free medium directly into the medium containing 10% serum with simultaneous harvest of spent medium beginning at 230 hr, while the 80-13.6 hybridoma had

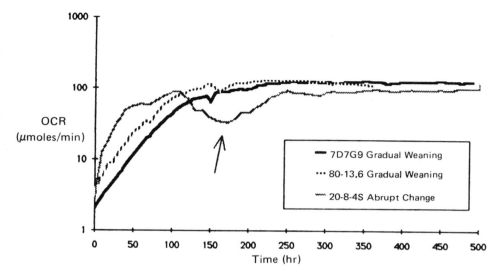

Figure 9 OCR of three cell lines demonstrating effects of gradual weaning of the cells from serum-containing to serum-free medium. The cell lines were initiated in medium containing 10% serum. At 100 hr the 20-8-4S line was batch changed to serum-free medium, followed by continuous feed and harvest. This rapid switch resulted in a drop in the OCR, as indicated by the arrow. 7D7G9 and 80-13.6 both had continuous feed and harvest with serum-free medium added directly into the medium containing serum at 190 hr and 164 hr, respectively. This allowed for gradual serum reduction, and showed no drop in OCR.

continuous feed of serum-free medium into the medium containing serum starting at 160 hr. This procedure allowed for a gradual removal of serum from both the cultures, unlike the initial batch change shown with the 20-8-4S line. This gradual removal eliminated the drop in OCR, as was seen in the rapid switch. It could allow a particularly sensitive cell line to be easily adapted to serum free medium with a minimum of problems.

Several reports have discussed how a culture can be affected by oxygen levels (14-17). The antibody production can also be increased by changing the dissolved oxygen titer available to the culture. Figure 10 shows the OCR and antibody concentration of the hybridoma culture 20-8-4S maintained in the OPTICELL. This culture was grown for 3 days in RPMI 1640 with 10% FBS, then changed to 20 L modified Iscoves medium with 1% FBS for 2 days, followed by continuous feed and harvest of the modified Iscoves with

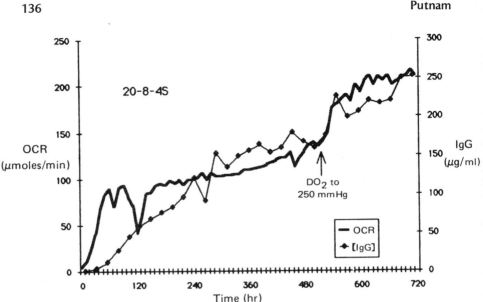

Figure 10   Correlation between O_2 titer and OCR and IgG concentration with 20-8-4S cell line in 1% FBS. At 520 hr, the O_2 in was changed from 145 to 250 mmHg. Both OCR and IgG concentration increased dramatically.

1% FBS at the rate of 11 L/day. The partial pressure of oxygen entering the culture was maintained at 145 mmHg (i.e., standard atmospheric oxygen level) for the first 520 hr of the culture. Then the level was raised to approximately 250 mmHg (i.e., 170% atmospheric oxygen level) for the remainder of the culture. During the time of continuous feed and harvest, at 145 mmHg oxygen, the OCR rose slowly from 100 to approximately 140. When the oxygen level was raised by 70% the OCR increased by 40% within 70 hr. But of more interest was that the concentration of antibody in the medium rose by about 25% after the oxygen levels were increased, reaching approximately 240 μg/ml. This implies that the level of oxygen is one of many ways that should be used to maximize production for a particular cell line. It is effective and does not impose any additional costs due to increased medium usage. The above results indicate that oxygen deficiency could be the limiting factor for maximizing antibody production in many large scale systems.

    As indicated previously, the OPTICELL System has been used with many types of hybridomas, including human–human and human–mouse. The system is particularly useful with these type of cells, since often their productivity is quite low when conventional methods of production are used. The ability to monitor culture respiration combined with the use of continuous feed and harvest, and the ability to wean these often sensitive cells from a growth medium to a production medium, has proven to be very helpful in maximizing the amount of usable product gained during a run.

VI. COMMENTS

The OPTICELL Culture System utilizing a porous ceramic matrix as a growth chamber compares very favorably to other technologies currently in use. It offers the benefits of an immobilized culture, the ease of product removal without a corresponding removal of cells, and, most importantly, the ability to monitor and maximize antibody production utilizing the OCR of the culture. In addition, it offers the ability to determine optimal parameters for maximum antibody production, such as increasing the amount of oxygen to the culture or the use of continuous feed and harvest. One can also see the immediate effect of adding a different type of medium to the culture and wean cells easily from a growth medium to a production medium without shocking the culture. The size of the system can be scaled for whatever the needs of production, from a system that can run six matrices simultaneously to one using a matrix approximately one-fifth the size described in this chapter. One disadvantage of the ceramic matrix would be, however, that although it may produce a greater amount of product per total volume of medium used than other systems, it may not offer as high a final product concentration as seen with the semipermeable membranes or the hollow fibers. This has not been a major problem, especially given the excellent overall efficiency of the system, since it is easy to incorporate a concentration device into the downstream processing. Through the ceramic's ability to immobilize the culture, the simple design of the growth chamber, and the system's controlling features, along with the direct contact of medium over the cells, the OPTICELL Culture System provides a very effective and reliable method of large-scale monoclonal antibody production.

ACKNOWLEDGMENTS

I would like to thank Dr. Bjorn K. Lydersen for his excellent guidance and counsel during the development of the system's adaptation to hybridoma culture, and for supplying the HMB 109 cell line. I also thank Gordon G. Pugh for his excellent advice, Lee A. Noll and R. Michael Worley for their counsel in critically reviewing this manuscript, and Dr. Paul G. Abrams for supplying the 7D7G9 and 80-13.6 cell lines.

REFERENCES

1. Kennett, R. H. (1981). Hybridomas: A new dimension in biological analyses. *In Vitro 17*: 1036-1050.
2. Tolbert, W. R. and Feder, J. (1983). Large-scale cell culture technology. *Ann. Rep. Ferment. Pro. 6*: 35-74.
3. Jarvis, A. P. Jr. and Grdina, T. A. (1983). Production of biologicals from microencapsulated living cells. *BioTechniques 1*: 22-27.
4. Spier, R. E. (1980). Recent developments in the large scale cultivation of animal cells in monolayers. *Adv. Biochem. Engin. 14*: 119-162.
5. Seaver, S., Rudolph, J. L., Ducibella, T., and Gabriels, J. E. (1984). Hybridoma cell metabolism/antibody secretion in culture. *BIOTECH '84 USA*, Online Publications, pp. 325-345.
6. Knazek, R. A., Gullino, P. M., Kohler, P. O., and Dedrick, R. L. (1972). Cell culture on artificial capillaries: An approach to tissue growth in vitro. *Science 178*: 65-66.
7. Ku, K., Kuo, M. J., Delente, J., Wildi, B. S., and Feder, J. (1981). Development of a hollow-fiber system for large-scale culture of mammalian cells. *Biotechnol. Bioeng. 23*: 79-95.
8. Lydersen, B. K., Pugh, G. G., Paris, M. S., Sharma, B. P., and Noll, L. A. (1985). Ceramic matrix for large scale animal cell culture. *Bio/Technology 3*: 63-67.
9. Bognar, E. A., Pugh, G. G., and Lydersen, B. K. (1983). Large scale propagation of BHK_{21} cells using the OPTICELL culture system. *J. Tissue Cult. Methods. 8*: 147-154.
10. Berg, G. J. (1985). An integrated system for large scale cell culture. *Dev. Biol. Standard 60*: 297-303.
11. Bodeker, B. G. D. (1985). Einsatz des Opticell-Kultursystem. *Labor Praxis* Sept: 970-980.
12. Swartz, R. (1985). Alternatives for the production of mammalian cell products: A survey. *Gen. Eng. News. 5* (7): 16-21.
13. Abrams, P. G., Knost, J. A., Clarke, G., Wilburn, S., Oldham, R. K., and Foon, K. A. (1983). Determination of the optimal human cell lines for development of human hybridomas. *J. Immunol. 131*: 1201-1204.
14. Pace, D. M., Thompson, J. R., and Van Camp, W. A. (1962). Effects of oxygen on growth in several established cell lines. *J. Na. Cancer Inst. 28*: 897-909.
15. Stephenson, N. G. (1969). Effects of increased partial pressures of oxygen, nitrogen, and helium on cells in culture. *Cell Tissue Kinet. 2*: 225-234.
16. Gendimenico, G. J., Schlesinger, H. R., Ritter, M. A., and Haugaard, N. (1984). Inhibition of growth and decreased survival of B104 rat neuroblastoma cells after exposure to hyperbaric oxygen. *In Vitro 20*: 385-390.
17. Spier, R. E. and Griffiths, B. (1984). An examination of the data and concepts germane to the oxygenation of cultured animal cells. *Dev. Biol. Standard. 55*: 81-92.

8

Large-Scale Production and Purification of Monoclonal Antibodies Using Cellular Microencapsulation

ELIZABETH G. POSILLICO,* MICHAEL S. KALLELIS,† and
JEAN M. GEORGE‡
Damon Biotech, Needham Heights, Massachusetts

I. INTRODUCTION

Following the important development of hybridoma technology by Kohler and Milstein (1) in 1975, utilization of monoclonal antibodies in the health care field has grown dramatically. The unique advantages of monoclonal antibodies are that they have a single specificity and can be produced almost indefinitely using hybridoma cell culture.

Monoclonal antibodies have been used to discern the molecular differences between healthy and diseased cells and to study the agents that cause disease. Due to their unique and singular specificities, monoclonal antibodies are being studied extensively in clinical trials for their efficacy in the treatment of several diseases including a variety of cancers (2-5), transplant rejection (6), rhinovirus infection (7), and blood disorders (8).

As in vivo diagnostic imaging agents, monoclonal antibodies can be either radiolabeled or coupled to specific opaque dyes to allow physicians to identify and localize primary and metastatic tumors (9,10).

Present affiliation: Genzyme Corporation, Boston, Massachusetts.
†*Present affiliation*: Milligen Division, Millipore Corporation, Bedford, Massachusetts.
‡*Present affiliation*: Simmons College, Boston, Massachusetts.

139

Another important application of monoclonal antibodies is as reagents in in vitro diagnostic test kits. Since they are a homogenous preparation of immunoglobulin molecules, the immunochemical properties of monoclonal antibodies are consistent from lot to lot. This advantage eliminates the problems of lot-to-lot variability inherent in preparations of polyclonal antibodies.

With the rising demand for monoclonal antibodies, both in research investigations and in the commercial marketplace, the need for production systems and facilities to manufacture monoclonal antibodies on a large scale has increased. Mammalian cell culture techniques have been utilized for scientific research and vaccine production for many years, but their large-scale application to the production of biological products, such as monoclonal antibodies, is still very much in its infancy. As the need for biological products has increased, the research and development in mammalian cell culture technologies have also increased. Bacterial fermentation systems cannot be used for the commercial production of complex biological molecules such as monoclonal antibodies, tissue plasminogen activitor (tPA), viral antigens, and glycosylated peptide hormones. Such proteins require glycosylation, specific sulfide bond formation, or other posttranslational modifications for proper molecular conformation and activity (11).

While mammalian cell culture provides a solution for the production of complex biological compounds in vitro, cell culture systems have certain limitations and inherent problems that complicate their use on a large scale. Until recently, the major limitation of traditional cell culture was low cell densities and, therefore, low product yields. In recent years there has been a major commitment to the development of new mammalian cell culture methodologies to overcome the problems of low cell densities and low product concentrations. As a result, several novel cell culture techniques have been developed. These include the use of rotating perfusion filters (12), hollow fiber technology (13), ceramic matrices (14), airlift fermentors (15), and microencapsulation (16-19). At the production scale, significant differences among cell culture technologies can be appreciated more from the impact that they have upon downstream processing and purification of product than from their ability to support cell growth and produce product.

The following discussion will focus on the use of the ENCAPCEL microencapsulation process for the production of monoclonal antibodies on a large scale and the methods used for downstream processing and purification of product. The microencapsulation process, originally described by Dr. Franklin Lim, encases cells in a semipermeable polymer membrane (20). Damon Biotech introduced its patented encapsulation process, ENCAPCEL, in 1982. Over the past three years, this technology has been successfully taken from a research scale to a production scale. Microencapsulation is now routinely used for the commercial manufacture of large quantities of monoclonal antibodies used in diagnostic testing assays, large-scale industrial purification procedures, and in vivo diagnostic imaging and cancer therapy (17–19).

II. MICROENCAPSULATION SYSTEM

A. Microcapsule Formation

Microencapsulation is a novel cell culture process that encases cells inside a semipermeable biopolymer membrane. This is accomplished by first immobilizing cells in sodium alginate gel spheres, coating the spheres with a specific biopolymer to make the capsule membrane, and finally reliquifying the interior gel. The process is shown diagramatically in Figure 1.

The ENCAPCEL method of microencapsulation is a mild chemical process that uses isotonic aqueous solutions, physiological pH, operating temperatures between 20 and 37°C, and biocompatible membrane constituents. The entire process is completed in approximately 2½ hr. As a result of these mild conditions, microencapsulation of hybridoma cells does not compromise growth potential, cell viability, or the synthesis of specific cellular products.

To prepare the gel spheres, hybridoma cells are mixed with sodium alginate at an initial seeding density of 2×10^6 cells/ml, a density close to the maximum density attainable with traditional suspension culture. The cell/alginate suspension is passed through a droplet-forming apparatus, and the droplets are gelled by contact with a dilute solution of calcium chloride. The gel spheres are then sterilely transferred to a 40 L bioreactor, where the semipermeable membrane is layered onto the periphery of the gel spheres by stepwise addition of reagents including a polycationic, polyamino acid compound that binds to the alginate spheres through salt bond formation. When microcapsule formation is complete, a brief exposure to a chelating agent reliquifies the intracapsular alginate. Reliquification allows cells to migrate within the microcapsule and facilitates the diffusion of nutrient medium. Within each encapsulation run, microcapsules do not vary in size by more than about 15%, and typical microcapsule diameters used in our production runs range from 700 to 900 μm. Immediately following encapsulation, culture medium is added to the bioreactor, and the encapsulated cells are cultured at 37°C for 2–4 weeks.

The permeability of the microcapsule membrane can be varied to suit the specific application. In the case of monoclonal IgG production from hybridoma cells, the permeability of the microcapsule is adjusted to allow for diffusion of albumin and other proteins with molecular weights up to approximately 90,000 daltons, but to constrain the IgG (150,000 daltons) within the microcapsule. Control of membrane permeability is determined by the concentration of the polycations, their molecular weight, and the reaction time of the coating process. The benefits of antibody retention

1. Formation of Gel Spheres

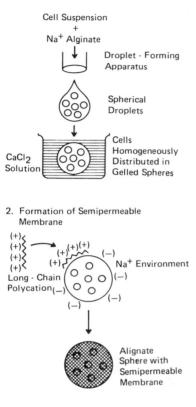

2. Formation of Semipermeable
   Membrane

3. Growth of Microencapsulated
   Cell Cultures

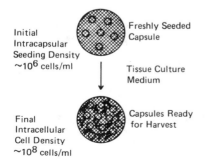

Figure 1   The microencapsulation process.

within the microcapsules are high product concentration, high starting purity, no detectable contamination of product with nonspecific serum immunoglobulins, and the ability to process product in discrete batches. All of these features simplify and streamline downstream processing and purification.

B. Culture Conditions and Controls

For the production of monoclonal antibodies, encapsulated cultures are maintained for 2-4 weeks, at which time the antibody is ready to be harvested. Typically, 6 L of microcapsules are cultured in 25 L of medium. Microcapsule cultures are continuously supplied with media throughout the culture period at a rate dependent upon cell density. The total volume of media used for supporting cell growth in microcapsules is comparable to that required for traditional cell suspension methods.

The microcapsule cultures are sampled periodically to determine total cell number and percent viability. A unique advantage of microencapsulation is that the cells are protected inside the microcapsule. Under these conditions, microcapsules can be stirred at much higher rates than suspension cultures; this improves both nutrient and gas exchange, and, in contrast to traditional cell suspension, cells are not subjected to shear forces, which can compromise cell viability (21,22).

The micrographs in Figure 2 show the growth pattern of a murine hybridoma cell line during a 3-week culture period. Immediately following the encapsulation process, cells are at an approximate density of 2×10^6 cells/ml and are evenly distributed within the microcapsules. By day 5 of culture, cell number has increased to 1×10^7 cells/ml microcapsules, and there are large foci of cell growth located primarily near the periphery of the microcapsules. By day 10-12, the total cell number has reached $2-4 \times 10^7$ cells/ml, and by day 15 to 20, $4 \times 10^7-1 \times 10^8$ cells/ml. Encapsulated cells grow preferentially near the interior surface of the microcapsules where nutrient exchange is greatest. By the end of the culture period, the cells form a tissuelike layer that covers roughly three-quarters of the interior capsule surface. Cell densities increase approximately 50-100-fold in a typical capsule culture (Fig. 3). Final concentrations of antibody range from 0.5 to 3 mg/ml capsules depending upon the cell line and its rate of antibody production (Fig. 3). At these concentrations, 5-20 g antibody is currently being produced by one 40 L fermentor. Higher product yields from the bioreactors are expected in the future as a result of continuing improvements in the encapsulation process, as well as industry-wide advances in cell culture techniques and improvements in bioreactor operation and design. Since the production of biological products on a large scale is a relatively new field, the biotechnology industry has a lot to learn before current cell culture methods can be considered fully optimized.

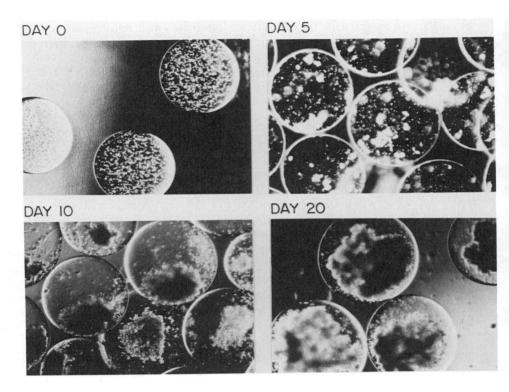

Figure 2 Photomicrographs of hybridoma cell growth in capsules. Photographs were taken of cell growth in capsules on days 0, 5, 10, 20 of culture. The initial density of cells in capsules is about 1×10^6/ml of capsules and after 20 days in culture, total cell density ranges from 3×10^7 to 1×10^8/ml.

Experience has shown that both cell growth and antibody production are highly dependent upon the hybridoma line. A cell line's performance in microcapsules, however, does correlate with its growth and antibody production characteristics in suspension culture. Hybridomas that produce well in suspension culture generally produce well in microcapsules. Over 80 different hybridoma cell lines (of both mouse and rat origin) have been grown in microcapsules, and all of them have produced multiple-gram quantities of monoclonal antibody, including rat IgG and mouse IgG, IgA, and IgM.

An important aspect of any production system is to have control over that system: over critical materials and equipment as well as production procedures. Dependence upon an outside vendor for critical process equipment

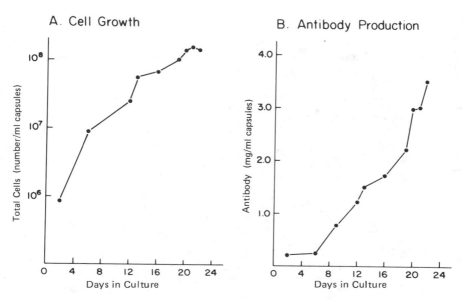

Figure 3   A: Hybridoma cell growth in microcapsules. B: Antibody production in microcapsules. Data for A and B are from the same capsule culture. These demonstrate the rapid cell growth in microcapsules over a 20-day culture period and the concomitant increase in intracapsular antibody concentration during this same time.

or compounds can result in significant delays. if vendors experience their own manufacturing problems or delays. Thus three important components of the cell culture process are produced in-house. First, bioreactors have been developed and designed to meet the needs of microcapsule culture (Fig. 4). These have been designed specifically to simplify operation and facilitate bioreactor maintenance and repair in-house. Substantial time delays can be encountered waiting for an outside vendor to service fermentation equipment. Second, the biopolymers necessary to make the microcapsule membrane are produced in-house, thereby ensuring the capability and the flexibility to keep pace with increasing production needs. Third, the large volume of media required for a production-scale mammalian cell culture process is produced in-house.

Quality control over the procedures required for the production of monoclonal antibodies is accomplished using a standardized, optimized encapsulation process that is conducted using current Good Manufacturing Practices (cGMPs). One production process is now used for all monoclonal antibody

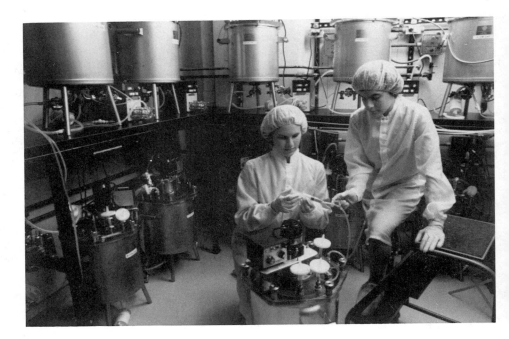

Figure 4   The 40 L bioreactors used for culturing microcapsules.

production. Monoclonal antibodies have been prepared from over 80 different hybridoma cell lines using the same culture medium, the same culture conditions, and the same encapsulation process for each. Experience has shown that media and culture conditions do not necessarily have to be optimized for each individual cell line. For the contract production of antibody from many different hybridomas, the time spent optimizing the culture conditions for slight potential improvements in cell growth and antibody production is better spent in producing the product itself. Moreover, on a production scale, it is particularly important to keep the media costs at a minimum. Accordingly, increased serum concentrations and growth factors that may provide slight improvements in antibody production are generally not cost-effective. However, if a product is to be produced over a long period of time (>6 months), optimization of culture conditions clearly becomes more valuable in terms of cost benefits over the long term.

Culture medium to be used in a manufacturing process deserves some discussion, since considerable amounts of complex culture media must be manufactured in any large scale cell culture facility. The productivity and efficiency of a large scale media preparation laboratory are hampered significantly if several different media formulations must be prepared. Fortunately, since monoclonal antibody is constrained within the microcapsule membrane, serum can be used to supplement the culture medium without contaminating the monoclonal antibody with nonspecific immunoglobulins. Serum not only promotes growth of most hybridomas but also appears to be required for the growth of certain lines. A modified formulation of Williams Medium E developed in-house and supplemented with 5% horse serum is used exclusively in the production facility (23). The basal medium is more enriched than conventional culture media and therefore costs are somewhat higher; however, this medium has been successfully used to support continuous growth of over 100 different hybridoma cell lines from mouse, rat, and human origin as well as several other nonhybridoma cell lines. There is no significant difference in either cell growth or antibody production between cells grown in media supplemented either with horse serum or fetal calf serum at 5% and 10%. Horse serum is not only one-third the cost of fetal calf, but also is obtained from donor herds that provide more lot-to-lot consistency. The supplemented medium used in-house is one-third to one-fifth the cost of commercially available serum-free formulations. With several different cell lines in production simultaneously, the use of one culture medium greatly increases medium production capacity and efficiency.

III. CONSIDERATIONS AND PROBLEMS RELATED TO LARGE-SCALE ANTIBODY PURIFICATION

The purification process is the most difficult aspect of a commercial antibody production process to standardize. The unique biological specificities of monoclonal antibodies are based upon subtle molecular differences. The biochemical nature of these differences may or may not alter the conditions required for purification. An antibody's subclass, its isoelectric point, and its stability at different pHs are factors known to influence the selection of a purification technique. The difficulty for the contract producer is that in most cases the biochemical properties of each specific immunoglobulin are unknown, and considerable time and effort can be spent conducting pilot studies to define them. Particularly in the purification process, some standardization of methods is essential to produce multiple antibody products in an efficient and cost-effective manner.

Both the initial purity and the specific types of contaminants present in crude antibody preparations affect the selection of purification techniques. Previous standardization of the cell culture process greatly simplifies the purification scheme, because contaminating proteins remain constant from one lot to the next. Therefore, when a purification process has been developed that can remove the unwanted proteins, the only variable among antibody lots is the antibody itself. It should be apparent, then, that variations in the composition of cell culture media for the optimization of cell growth may cause problems and delays during purification.

One of the factors that complicates purification of antibodies produced in ascites or cell suspension is the presence of nonspecific immunoglobulins introduced into the product by either the mouse host or the serum used to supplement the culture media. Failure to remove these immunoglobulin contaminants reduces the specific activity of a monoclonal antibody. Unfortunately, the presence of nonspecific immunoglobulins may preclude the use of ion exchange chromatography as the sole purification method because the nonspecific antibodies copurify with the desired monoclonal antibody. Affinity chromatography, using specific antigens, obviates this problem; however, this purification method suffers from two disadvantages. First, the resins are costly and have to be custom-made. Second, the elution conditions required for affinity purification, such as low pH, can cause considerable reduction in the activity of certain antibodies (18,24). Therefore, activity assays and specific purification procedures for each product have to be developed and implemented by the contract producer to prevent inactivation of the antibody.

Protein A is an alternative method for purification of immunoglobulins that results in high purity levels. However, protein A chromatography also requires reduced pH for elution, which may reduce biological activity. In addition, the affinity of protein A for the various subclasses of immunoglobulin varies considerably. For example, human and certain mouse IgG3 antibodies do not bind to protein A, and the degree to which mouse IgG1 binds tends to vary (25). Since IgG1 and IgG2a subclasses form the majority of murine monoclonal antibodies, this method is neither reliable or universal.

Table 1 compares the activity of one monoclonal antibody following purification by ion exchange and by antigen specific affinity chromatography. In the latter case, elution of the antibody with an acetate buffer resulted in high recovery, but antibody activity dropped 67%. Antibody activity improved slightly when a glycine/HCl elution buffer was used, but recovery was greatly diminished (to only 33%). Ion exchange, on the other hand, gave both high levels of activity (>99%) and very good recovery (95%).

Another important consideration is the capability for scale-up of a chosen purification technique. For example, two factors that can be prohibitive for large-scale purification using HPLC are the current limited capacity of preparative columns for purification of gram quantities of product and the expense of equipment required to run large-scale HPLC systems. Similarly, the

Table 1 Intracapsular Antibody Activity Following Purification by Affinity Versus Ion Exchange Chromatography

	Antibody activity (%)	Recovery (%)	Final purity (%)
Affinity chromatography			
Acetate	32	93	>98
Glycine HCl	52	33	>98
Ion exchange	>99	95	>98

Intracapsular antibody was purified by passing it over a DEAE, Tris-acryl (LKB-Produkter, Sweden) column or over an affinity column to which the antigen to the antibody was covalently coupled. Bound antibody was eluted from the affinity matrix with either 0.1 M acetic acid (pH 2.8) or 0.1 M glycine/HCl (pH 2.5) and collected into tubes containing a Tris pH 7.5 buffer to minimize denaturation of the antibody. The activity of purified antibody, prepared by either ion-exchange or affinity column, was determined by passing purified antibody over the antigen–affinity column and eluting with 0.1 M acetic acid. Total antibody protein recovered from the column was determined by the method of Lowry, et al. The activity was estimated as total antibody protein bound to the affinity column divided by total antibody placed on the column × 100% (from ref. 18 with permission.)

preparation of antigen-specific affinity resins is readily carried out in a research laboratory, but in a commercial production facility the preparation of a special affinity resin for each antibody is clearly not cost-effective. Preparation of the purification media would probably exceed the time required to produce the antibody.

IV. PURIFICATION OF INTRACAPSULAR ANTIBODY

Standardized large-scale purification of intracapsular antibody has been achieved because of two advantages of the microencapsulation production system: high starting purity of crude product and lot-to-lot reproducibility. Intracapsular antibody prior to purification has an unusually high purity ranging from 45 to 80%, depending on the productivity of each cell line.

In preparation for purification, intracapsular antibodies may be concentrated by either ammonium sulfate precipitation or ultrafiltration. Historically, ammonium sulfate precipitation of antibody preparations has been necessary not only as a concentration step but also as an intermediate purification step. However, with the high starting purity of antibody produced by

microencapsulation, recent studies have shown that the ammonium sulfate
precipitation step is not necessary as an intermediate purification step and
can be eliminated. This precipitation procedure is not only time-consuming
and difficult to perform on a large scale, but it also can result in antibody
losses of 10–25%. Furthermore, certain antibodies have been identified,
especially of the IgM and IgG3 classes, that do not precipitate well using
ammonium sulfate.

Ultrafiltration is a good alternative, since this method can concentrate
large volumes of biological material in a fraction of the time required to concentrate using ammonium sulfate precipitation. Due to the fact that ultrafiltration is rapid and that the equipment can be easily depyrogenated, this
method of concentration is particularly useful for the preparation of therapeutic-grade products. Furthermore, the same equipment can be utilized
following the concentration step for diafiltration of product into the appropriate purification buffer.

Concentrated intracapsular antibody preparations are purified by ion-
exchange chromatography. Antibody purities in excess of 98% of total protein are routinely achieved following one pass over an ion exchange column.
The various process steps currently used to purify intracapsular antibody are
listed in Table 2. The right-hand column lists the testing procedures performed during the purification process. These tests, with the exception of
the pyrogen test, are performed on all antibodies in production. Pyrogen
testing is performed at each step of the purification procedure only for
therapeutic products or products that require validation of low pyrogen
levels. Immunoglobulin concentration is determined by a nephelometric immunoassay and by spectrophotometric absorbance at 280 nm. Typical
recoveries of antibody after ammonium sulfate precipitation and ion exchange
chromatography are shown in Table 3. The average recovery of antibody after
final purification of six separate preparations of product was 88.2%. Conductivity measurements are made to provide assurance that buffer exchange
is complete. SDS gel electrophoresis and HPLC using an ion exchange column
are methods used to determine product purity. Figure 5 demonstrates the
purity of three different preparations of purified therapeutic-grade antibody
as analyzed by SDS gel electrophoresis. The two bands of protein correspond
to the heavy and light chains of the immunoglobulin molecule. In lanes 5–7,
the two light chains produced by this hybridoma line can be clearly differentiated. Antibody purity of all preparations was determined to be >98%
by densitometric analysis of the Coomassie-blue-stained gel. Antibody purity
of final product is also analyzed by HPLC. Figure 6 is a typical chromatogram of final therapeutic product. Antibody purity was >99% using computerized peak integration.

Table 2 IgG Purification and Product Testing

Step	Tests performed
1. Crude intracapsular antibody	Ig concentration Pyrogens
2. Concentration	Ig concentration Pyrogens
3. Precipitation: 60% NH_4SO_4 [a]	Ig concentration Pyrogens

4. Diafiltration against ion exchange buffer	Product
	  pH
	  Conductivity
	  Ig concentration
	  Pyrogens
	Column
	  pH
	  Conductivity
	  Pyrogens

5. Ion exchange chromatography	Product
	  Ig concentration
	  Pyrogens
	  SDS gel electrophoresis
	  HPLC
	Column
	  pH
	  Conductivity
	  Pyrogens

6. Diafiltration against 0.9% NaCl	Ig concentration Pyrogens
7. Final bulk product analysis	Ig concentration DNA polynucleotide Mycoplasma Specificity HPLC

Table 2   (Continued)

Step	Tests performed
7. Final bulk product analysis (continued)	SDS gel electrophoresis
	Pyrogens
	Total protein
8. Final vialed product analysis	Sterility
	Ig subclass
	Ig concentration
	General safety
	Particulates
	Pyrogens
	Total protein

[a]Step 3 can be eliminated.

Ion-exchange chromatography has several advantages over affinity methods (e.g., antigen-specific resins and protein A). First, ion exchange is an established technique conducted using mild physiological conditions that do not compromise antibody activity. Second, ion-exchange resins have a high binding capacity for many types of contaminants including bacterial endotoxins. The ability to remove pyrogens provides additional quality assurance in the preparation of therapeutic grade products. Third, the process is cost-effective and can be readily scaled-up to accommodate production scale demands. Finally, this method is an accepted technique from a regulatory standpoint and is currently used worldwide on a production scale for the purification of several other pharmaceutical products.

An acrylic DEAE resin has been used very successfully. The acrylic-type media have good flow rates and are resistant to compaction, which makes them particularly well-suited to large-scale applications. The same resin and purification protocol may be used to purify 50 mg or 50 g. Ion-exchange media have been particularly useful for the preparation of therapeutic product, because they can be depyrogenated readily by brief exposure to 0.1 M NaOH and stored in 50% ethanol. Using sterile, depyrogenated protein processing and purification equipment, low pyrogen levels are maintained throughout the purification procedure (see Table 4).

Table 3 Antibody Recovery During Purification

Antibody lot	Initial crude antibody (g)	Recovery after ammonium sulfate		Recovery after chromatography	
		g	%	g	%
850311	9.2	7.8	84.7	7.2	78.3
850312	10.5	8.8	83.8	7.6	72.3
850403	4.2	4.6	100.0	4.7	100.0
850411	20.0	18.7	93.5	18.2	93.5
850508	14.0	13.9	99.2	13.6	97.1
860102	24.3	26.7	100.0	21.3	87.7
Average			93.5		88.2

Antibody recovery from six separate preparations of product was evaluated following ammonium sulfate precipitation and ion exchange chromatography. The average recovery after ammonium sulfate precipitation was 93.5%. Total average recovery following ammonium sulfate precipitation and ion exchange chromatography was 88.2%. Antibody concentration was measured using a nephelometric immunoassay with subclass-specific standards.

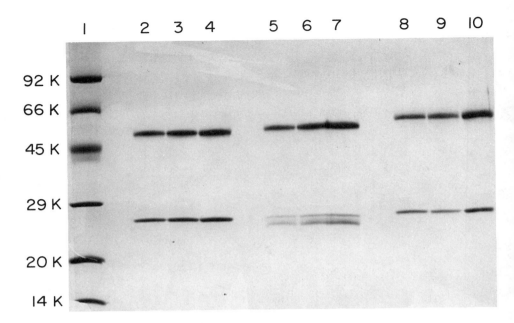

Figure 5 SDS gel electrophoresis of purified intracapsular antibody. Three separate monoclonal antibodies (MAbs) purified by DEAE ion exchange chromatography were analyzed by SDS gel electrophoresis under reducing conditions using a 10-20% gradient gel. For each preparation, samples of 7.5, 10, and 12.5 μg were loaded on the gels (MAb 1: lanes 2-4; MAb 2: lanes 5-7; MAb 3: lanes 8-10). Molecular weight standards were run in lane 1. Purity of each monoclonal antibody was determined to be >98% by densitometric analysis of the gel stained with Coomassie blue.

Table 4   Pyrogen Analysis of Antibody Product

Antibody lot	Unpurified Ab		Purified final product	
	Ab concentration (mg/ml)	Pyrogens (eu/ml)	Ab concentration (mg/ml)	Pyrogens (eu/ml)
841024	0.8	3.8-7.7	6.6	1.9-3.8
850926	2.6	1.5-3.0	1.3	1.5-3.0
851120	2.2	0.15-1.5	4.7	2.4-4.8
860108	3.7	6.0-12.0	3.6	2.4-4.8

Total pyrogen levels in four separate preparations of antibody product were measured in unpurified antibody and in purified antibody following ion exchange chromatography. Total pyrogens as measured by the LAL limulus amebocyte assay were <5 eu/ml in all final product analyzed.

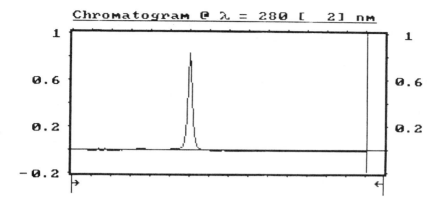

Figure 6 Analysis of purified intracapsular antibody by HPLC chromatography. Purified therapeutic-grade antibody was analyzed using a Waters
DEAE-5TW column equilibrated with 20 mM Tris buffer. Samples were
eluted with a NaCl gradient of 0–300 mM over 1 hr at a flow rate of 1 ml/
min. A computerized system for peak integration showed antibody purity to
be >98%.

V. SUMMARY

The ENCAPCEL cellular microencapsulation process has been standardized
and optimized for the large-scale production of monoclonal antibodies. The
ENCAPCEL process has several advantages that make it especially useful for
manufacturing facilities. In particular, the high intracapsular antibody concentrations and purities reached within 20 days of culture represent an
economy of scale unrivaled by several other technologies currently used to
produce monoclonal antibodies. In addition, serum-supplemented media can
be used without complicating downstream purification of product. Finally,
due to high starting purity, intracapsular antibody can be purified to greater
than 98% by ion-exchange chromatography. This method is simple, can be
scaled-up easily, and does not compromise antibody activity. Antibodies
produced by microencapsulation are being utilized in diagnostic assays, in
large-scale purification of biologicals, and for in vivo imaging and the treatment of human cancer and other diseases.

REFERENCES

1. Kohler, G. and Milstein, C. (1975). Continuous cultures of fused cells
    secreting antibody of predefined specificity. *Nature 256*: 495.

2. Varki, N. M., Reisfeld, R. A., and Walker, L. E. (1984). Antigens associated with a human lung adenocarcinoma defined by monoclonal antibodies. *Cancer Res. 44*: 681–687.

3. Miller, R. A., Maloney, D. G., Warnke, R., and Levy, R. (1982). Treatment of B-cell lymphoma with monoclonal anti-idiotype antibody. *N. Engl. J. Med. 306*: 517–522.

4. Larson, S. M., Carrasquillo, J. A., Krohn, K. A., Brown, J. P., McGuffin, R. W., Fereno, J. M., Graham, M. M., Hill, L. D., Beaumier, P. L., Hellstrom, K. E., and Hellstrom, I. (1983). Localization of ^{131}I-labeled p97-specific Fab fragments in human melanoma as a basis for radiotherapy. *J. Clin. Invest. 72*: 2101–2114.

5. Foon, K. A., Schroff, R. W., Bunn, P. A., Mayer, D., Abrams, P. G., Fer, M., Ochs, J., Bottino, G. C., Sherwin, S. A., and Carlo, D. J. (1984). Effects of monoclonal antibody therapy in patients with chronic lymphocytic leukemia. *Blood 64*: 1085–1093.

6. Goldstein, G., Schindler, J., Tsai, H. et al. (1985). Ortho Multicenter Transplant Study group. A randomized clinical trial of OKT-3 monoclonal antibody for acute rejection of cadaveric renal transplants. *N. Engl. J. Med. 313*: 337–342.

7. Colonna, R. J., Callahan, P. L., and Long, W. J. (1986). Isolation of monoclonal antibody that blocks attachment of the major group of human rhinoviruses. *J. Virol. 57*: 7–12.

8. Clarkson, S. B., Bussel, J. B., Kimberly, R. P., Valinsky, J. E., Nachman, R. L., and Unkeless, J. C. (1986). Treatment of refractory immune thrombocytopenic purpura with an anti-FC receptor antibody. *N. Engl. J. Med. 314*: 1236–1239.

9. Larson, S. M., Brown, J. P., Wright, P. W., Carrasquillo, J. A., Hellstrom, I., and Hellstrom, K. E. (1983). Imaging of melanoma with I-131-labeled monoclonal antibodies. *J. Nucl. Med. 24*: 123–129.

10. Hnatowich, D. J., Griffin, T. W., Kosciuczyk, C., Rusckowski, M., Childs, R. L., Mattis, J. A., Shealy, D., and Doherty, P. W. (1985). Pharmacokinetics of an indium-111-labeled monoclonal antibody in cancer patients. *J. Nucl. Med. 26*: 849–858.

11. Berman, P. W., Gregory, T., Crase, D., and Laskey, L. (1985). Protection from genital herpes simplex virus type 2 infection by vaccination with cloned type 1 glycoprotein D. *Science 227*: 1490–1492.

12. Feder, J. and Tolbert, W. R. (1985). Mass culture of mammalian cells in perfusion systems. American Biotechnology Laboratory, January/February: 24–36.

13. Hopkinson, J. (1985). Hollow fiber cell culture systems for economical cell product manufacturing. *Biotechnology 3*: 225–230.

14. Lydersen, B. K., Pugh, G. C., Paris, M. S., Sharma, B. P., and Noll, L. A. (1985). Ceramic matrix for large scale animal cell culture. *Biotechnology 3*: 63–67.

15. Birch, J. R., Thompson, P. W., Lambert, K., and Boraston, R. (1985). The large scale cultivation of hybridoma cells producing monoclonal antibodies. In *Large-Scale Mammalian Cell Culture.* Edited by W. R. Tolbert and J. Feder. New York, Academic Press.
16. Duff, R. G. (1985). Microencapsulation technology: A novel method for monoclonal antibody production. *Trends Biotechnology 3*: 167–170.
17. Posillico, E. G. (1986). Microencapsulation technology for large-scale antibody production. *Biotechnology 4*: 114–117.
18. Rupp, R. (1985). Use of cellular microencapsulation in large-scale production of monoclonal antibodies. In *Large-Scale Mammalian Cell Culture.* Edited by W. R. Tolbert and J. Feder. New York, Academic Press, pp. 97–123.
19. Jarvis, A. P. Jr. and Grdina, T. A. (1983). Production of biologicals from microencapsulated living cells. *Biotechniques 1*: 22–37.
20. Lim, F. (1984). Microencapsulation of living cells and tissues—theory and practice. In *Biomedical Applications of Microencapsulation.* Edited by F. Lim. Boca Raton, CRC Press, pp. 137–154.
21. Augenstein, D. C., Sinskey, A. J., and Wang, D. I. C. (1971). Effect of shear on the death of two strains of mammalian tissue cells. *Biotechnol. Bioeng. 13*: 409–418.
22. Fazekas de St. Groth, S. (1983). Automated production of monoclonal antibodies in a cytostat. *J. Immunol. Methods 57*: 121–136.
23. Rupp, R. and Geyer, S. (1984). Preparation of medium for large scale hybridoma culture. *J. Tissue Culture Methods 8*: 141–145.
24. Ey, P. L., Prowse, S. J., and Jenkin, C. R. (1978). Isolation of pure IgG, IgG2a and IgG2b immunoglobulins from mouse serum using protein A-sepaharose. *Immunochemistry 15*: 429–436.
25. Hudson, L. and Hay, F. (1980). Affinity chromatography. In *Practical Immunology.* Oxford, Blackwell Scientific Publications, pp. 203–225.

9

Mass Culture of Mouse and Human Hybridoma Cells in Hollow-Fiber Culture

RANDALL J. VON WEDEL*
Bio-Response, Inc., Hayward, California

I. PRINCIPLES OF CONTINUOUS PERFUSION CELL CULTURE

A. Homeostasis

Simulation of the in vivo environment has always been a major and, at times, elusive goal of any cell culture system. Unlike conventional stirred tank (1), encapsulation (2,3) and airlift (4,5) culture systems, a continuous perfusion cell culture system allows for the perpetual removal of waste products and the uninterrupted replenishment of essential nutrients necessary for optimal production. In the approach taken by Bio-Response, the exchange of metabolites and nutrients is accomplished by infusion of fresh media combined with various configurations of external dialysis loops composed of selective semipermeable membranes. Careful monitoring of physiological parameters permits fine-tuned regulation of the composition and flow rates of medium through the various dialysis circuits. When coupled with the continuous harvest of secreted antibody and the regular removal of excess cells, this process control can maintain a state of homeostasis, providing uniform growth conditions over much longer periods of time than can be obtained with any batch-type process in which cells are subjected to the stress of exhausted medium. There is now an increasing trend in the industry to apply continuous perfusion culture practices to several other existing cell culture technologies (6-8; see other chapters in this book). Hence, continuous perfusion cell

---

Present affiliation: CytoCulture International, Inc., San Francisco, California.

culture is becoming more of an operational term than a description for a particular bioreactor design.

B. High Cell Density

One immediate benefit of a stabilized perfusion cell culture environment is that it promotes the growth of cells to higher densities than can be achieved with normal static culture or batch bioreactors. Typically, viable cell densities of 2-5 × 10^7 cells/ml can be maintained (usually with the aid of routine cell drains) in suspension cultures for weeks or months. High cell density not only increases the cost effectiveness of the system when large quantities of antibody are required but also greatly improves the initial purity of the antibody harvested from the units.

C. High Initial Purity

The combination of high cell densities and low protein concentrations of chemically defined media can result in the harvest of antibody at relatively high levels of purity. The constant replenishment of critical protein growth factors avoids the need to add high concentrations of protein supplements to the initial medium. Purity is further enhanced by the continual removal of low-molecular-weight contaminants. Hence, reports of initial antibody purities in the range of 50-70% from continuous perfusion culture systems are not uncommon for murine hybridomas.

D. Continuous Recovery of Antibody

Concomitant with the removal of metabolites and the infusion of nutrients, circulation of medium through selective permeable membrane systems permits the continuous harvesting of secreted antibody product. Harvested material is immediately transferred to a low-temperature environment for downstream processing, thus minimizing any degradation of antibody that might have occurred by prolonged exposure to cell culture supernatants at 37°C. In addition, the continual removal of antibody precludes any possible deleterious feedback inhibition phenomena and minimizes the losses should mechanical failure or microbial contamination occur.

II. IMPLEMENTATION OF MASS CULTURING TECHNIQUES

A. Semipermeable Membrane Technology

At Bio-Response, continuous perfusion cell culture is optimized by selected bioreactor configurations, suitable low-protein media, the delivery of oxygen, the dialysis of metabolites, and the harvest and concentration of antibody product. Similar applications of hollow-fiber, membrane, or artificial capillary technologies to mammalian cell culture are now evident in the literature (9–12) and in the industry (7).

B. Mass Culturing Technique Components

The mass culturing technique (MCT) system for hybridoma cells consists of one or more bioreactor core hollow fiber units, oxygenators, and pumps in a configuration that permits efficient delivery of nutrients and gases. The hollow fiber units and their associated hardware are modular and can be replaced or combined to augment a function without compromising the entire production run. The hollow fibers themselves are purchased from commercial suppliers, but most units are designed and fabricated at Bio-Response, or manufactured to their specifications by subcontractors. All components are carefully washed, tested under pressure, and then irradiated before the final system is installed in the 37°C culture room. The culture room is flanked by parallel cold rooms, one supplying the fresh media, the other for collecting the harvested cell products.

Figure 1 is a schematic representation of the MCT system in a configuration used for suspension cells such as hybridomas.

The growth chamber, here drawn conceptually as a box with a double line around it, is in fact a cylindrical hollow-fiber unit resembling conventional hollow-fiber dialysis cartridges. The viable cells are maintained in the extra-capillary space surrounding the fibers. The hollow-fiber capillaries running through the center of the chamber deliver a constant influx of freshly oxygenated medium supplemented with low levels of defined protein components selected to optimize production of antibody (determined by prior cell characterization studies). The hollow fibers are composed of a microporous membrane material, typically with a 0.2 μm diameter pore size to maximize diffusion of fresh nutrients.

The oxygenators for these units are silicon-rubber-based aerators. Oxygenation of cells in the growth chamber occurs through diffusion of oxygen-rich medium out of the lumen of the hollow fibers and into the growth chamber (i.e., extracapillary space). Simultaneously, oxygen-depleted medium diffuses out of the growth chamber and into the lumen of the hollow fibers. Appropriate dissolved oxygen tension is restored upon passage through the oxygenators.

The dialysis circuit, represented in Figure 1 as the product exclusion membrane (PXM), is an ultrafiltration hollow-fiber membrane dialysis loop that continuously removes low-molecular-weight metabolites and waste products from the growth chamber, while simultaneously restoring low-molecular-weight

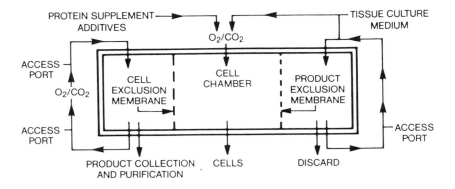

Figure 1 Schematic diagram of the mass culture system for hybridoma cultures at Bio-Response.

components such as vitamins and amino acids. High-molecular-weight cell products are retained within the dialysis loop because the membranes of the hollow fibers have a low-molecular-weight cut-off that varies from 5,000 to 10,000 MW. The dialysis loop is one of several control circuits regulated (changes in throughput volumes of medium, multiple units, etc.) as part of the process control program to maintain homeostasis within the system.

The product recovery circuit, represented in Figure 1 as the cell exclusion membrane (CXM), is a microporous membrane (0.2 μm) that allows cell-free antibody product to escape continually from the cell suspension in the extra-capillary space of the growth chamber. Although this process also depletes the cell suspension of needed protein supplements for growth, these factors are constantly being replenished by the infusion of fresh medium supplements into the extracapillary space of the growth chamber. Flow rates through the dialysis loop for the cell suspension from the growth chamber vary with the production rates of the cells. As the hybridoma culture matures, the volume of extracapillary dialysate may be increased to a maximum of around 10 L/day. The dialysate recycles through the product recovery loop until antibody concentrations approach around 100 μg/ml, at which point a portion of it is shunted to an adjacent refrigerated room for concentration with hollow-fiber or tangential flow concentrators.

Cell drains may be used to help maintain a productive environment. The number of cells removed and the frequency of drains are unique for each cell line. The cells are kept in suspension by continual rotation of the growth chamber. When used, the cell drains permit the MCT units to be maintained in a pseudocytostat mode of operation for long periods of time.

Analysis of the physiological parameters of each unit is accomplished by taking samples of medium or cell suspension at the various access ports indicated in Figure 1.

C. Customized Defined Media

The chemically defined medium for hybridoma cultures typically consists of a standard basal medium (e.g., 1:1 Dulbecco's Modified Eagle's Medium/Coon's F-12) supplemented with the minimal levels of protein supplements tailored to optimize viability and maximize productivity. These supplements include but are not limited to human or bovine transferrin (5 μg/ml) and insulin (1 μg/ml). Specific fatty acids, albumin and beta-mercaptoethanol are optional ingredients. No antibiotics are used in the MCT media and all ingredients are made up in pyrogen-free, injection grade distilled, deionized water. Only the inexpensive (protein-free) basal medium (DMEM/F-12) is used to filter away metabolites in the dialysis circuit.

Substantial effort is being invested in the development of suitable low-protein media to optimize the production of secreted proteins under the constraints of each cell line, particularly since cell lines have been found to require low amounts of serum supplement. Different formulations might be required at different stages of the bioprocess, but total medium protein concentrations are usually maintained under 40 μg/ml. All basal media used at Bio-Response are prepared in-house; the facility has the capacity to provide 10,000 L of media per week.

D. Process Control

Samples of medium or cell suspensions taken from the various sampling ports are analyzed in a chemistry lab adjacent to the culture room. Lactic acid and glucose are used as general indicators of cell metabolism; viable cell counts and lactate dehydrogenase levels are used to monitor viability. As in an intensive care unit, the staff of this process control laboratory is ready to respond if there is a change in critical physiological parameters, cell viability, or antibody production levels.

These parameters are usually monitored along with the corresponding operator responses.

Parameter	Response
pH, oxygen, carbon dioxide	Alter gas composition, and gas flow rate
Lactic acid, glucose ammonia	Alter medium flow rates
Viable cell count, lactic dehydro-genase, relevant product	Cell drains, alter medium flow rate

While computer-automated control could be used to monitor and adjust several of these parameters, it is not possible to monitor all pertinent parameters at this time. Until reliable, long-lasting probes are available for measuring lactic acid, ammonia, glucose, and others, most of these functions will have to be analyzed manually. Even if these probes were available, culture units would still need to be sampled because reliable product-specific probes are unlikely to be developed in the near future. In the meantime, however, Bio-Response has developed a streamlined analysis system for rapid feedback of operating parameter data in order to respond to variations in the metabolic demands of the culture units.

E. Scale-Up

A modular hollow-fiber perfusion culture system such as the MCT is readily amenable to scale-up by increasing the number of growth chamber units in one assembly and integrating the appropriate satellite support function units. The real advantage of a continuous homeostatic system, however, is that it can be operated productively for months at a time with little more than the routine efforts of process control and media replenishment. Thus, the initial capital investment in materials and labor for assembling and loading an industrial scale unit can be amortized over the 4–5 months of production time typical for hybridomas. In one case, a unit (glass bead bioreactor, otherwise similar support circuitry) producing a secreted cell protein from a genetically engineered cell line remained productive for 1 year. Naturally, as each unit stabilizes and patterns of cell growth and antibody productivity become predictable trends (analyzed on spread sheets and with computer graphics), operators can be more efficient in process control, and the per day costs of production continue to drop. In the meantime, advanced bioreactor designs with continuous *daily* output in the range of 5–10 g secreted antibody are under consideration.

III. PRODUCTION OF MURINE MONOCLONAL ANTIBODIES

A. Cell Characterization Studies

The production of any cellular protein at Bio-Response begins with the adaptation of the cell line (in conventional tissue culture flasks) to a chemically defined medium by gradually lowering the serum content. The defined medium contains the minimal protein supplements necessary to maintain high viability and maximal secretion of product. For hybridomas, this medium typically contains well under 40 μg/ml total protein, whereas the concentration of antibody product in the harvested medium can exceed 100 μg/ml. Antibody product levels are assayed by subclass specific ELISA techniques as well as by functional, antigen-binding assays. Murine hybridoma cell lines often adapt to the defined media within a few weeks, and maintain their production levels near or at the levels observed in normal serum-supplemented tissue culture medium prior to adaptation. The characterization program at this stage includes optimization of growth factors, glucose, buffers, fatty acids, trace elements, and gassing consistent with high cell density in the MCT system. Generally, a minimum of two MCT system units is then seeded with the adapted cell lines. As the cell density begins to rise, dialysis flow rates and gassing are adjusted to match the net metabolic levels of the unit. Antibody levels become appreciable by day 10–14, at which time the flow rate is adjusted through the product recovery loop to maintain equilibrium antibody levels between 20 and 100 μg/ml, depending on the particular hybridoma cell line. Pilot runs usually last a minimal of 30 days to fine tune the process control; enough antibody is generated to test purification regimens and for thorough characterization of the immunoglobulin's functional activity. After evaluation of the results, the cell line is expanded.

B. Routine MCT Production Runs

Typical production runs for hybridomas run about 2–3 months to satisfy the requirements of most contracts. Optimization protocols gathered during the cell characterization study are incorporated into process control to minimize any major changes once a production run has commenced.

Figure 2 demonstrates the long-term production of a monoclonal antibody from a standard murine hybridoma cell line maintained in continuous perfusion culture for over 5 months. Antibody production followed a cyclic pattern commonly observed in these long-term cultures. Antibody yields

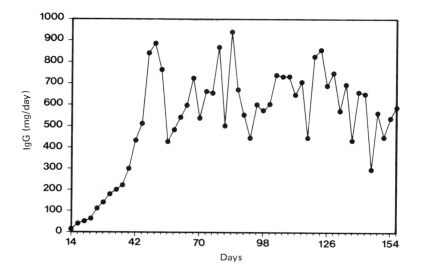

Figure 2   Monoclonal antibody production from a murine hybridoma: long-term continuous perfusion culture of murine hybridoma secreting IgG in chemically defined medium (MCT system using 800 ml capacity hollow-fiber growth chamber; total of 70 g/MAb produced from this single unit).

from this 1 L unit (extracapillary volume ~330 ml) averaged about 500–600 mg per day and totaled approximately 70 g when the unit was taken down. The average throughput of medium in the dialysate loop was 10 L. The defined medium used in this production run contained less than 50 μg/ml protein and average antibody levels in the harvested medium routinely exceeded that figure. This same cell line, grown in additional units, generated over 150 g functional monoclonal antibody at greater than 50% purity.

C. Downstream Processing

Harvested antibody product recovered from production culture units is accumulated in 20 L lots (often generated in less than 48 hours, depending on the product recovery flow rates.) Each lot is concentrated up to 50-fold on rapid, high-capacity ultrafiltration membrane concentrators (either of hollow fiber or tangential flow, flat sheet design) and assayed by ELISA. Lots are coded and tracked for the quality control department to ensure compliance with good manufacturing practices. The Bio-Response facility is fully capable of producing and handling materials for diagnostic or therapeutic applications; several of the antibodies produced in the MCT are destined for clinical trials.

Purification procedures depend on the quantity and end use classification of the antibody. The production process typically used at Bio-Response for monoclonal antibodies contributes to the purity of the product. Low-protein and defined media are preferentially used for therapeutic grade monoclonal antibodies. As mentioned above, cell exclusion membranes and rapid media throughputs minimize the period secreted product remains in the bioreactor and reduces contamination by cellular debris. With the use of this approach, a cell-free supernatant is aseptically collected in which well over 50% of the protein is the desired product. The advantage in purification of antibodies produced at greater than 50% of initial purity may be seen in Figure 3. A murine hybridoma cell line producing an IgG2a monoclonal antibody was grown and maintained for more than 4 months using the MCT process described previously. The antibody was produced in a defined medium known to contain approximately 50 μg/ml total protein. The antibody produced was analyzed on an 8.7% polyacrylamide gel with a 3% stacking gel prepared and run according to the standard Laemmli-denaturing gel procedure (19). Samples have been denatured with SDS buffer containing either iodoacetamide (lane 3,4,5) or B-mercaptoethanol (lane 1,7,9) and run on the same gel.

Lane 1 contains high- and low-molecular-weight standards. Lane 3 and 7 show purified standard murine IgG2a monoclonal antibody, treated with either IAM (lane 3) or BME (lane 7), respectively. The standard was purified using Protein A affinity chromatography. Lanes 4 and 8 show a concentrate of defined media, treated with either IAM or BME, respectively. Lanes 5 and 9 show the concentrated antibody containing cell-free supernatant collected from a MCT bioreactor, and treated with either IAM or BME, respectively. The cascade of lighter-staining bands present below the major antibody band, in both the standard lane 3 and the supernatant lane 5 are reactive with antimouse antibodies in general. They are most often thought to be glycosylation variants but many also reflect breakage of cells and partially assembled antibodies. These bands also appear when antibody is produced in ascites. The majority of the impurities in the antibody supernatant appear to be contributed by the defined media. A densitometric tracing of lane 5 revealed the following values

Major antibody band: 60.0%
Minor cascade: 11.0%
Transferrin: 15.0%
Minor band: 14.0%

Additional purification is tailored to the particular cell line and product. In general, ion exchange chromatography can be used to achieve purity levels of at least 95%. For some antibodies, additional chromatographic steps may

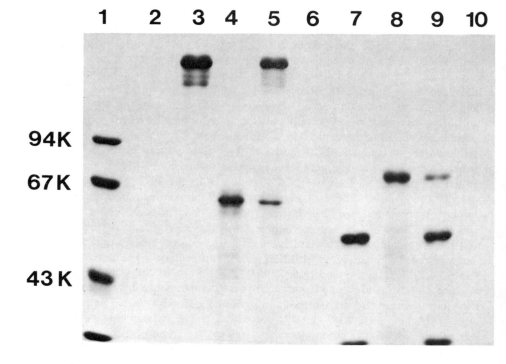

Figure 3 8.7% Polyacrylamide electrophoresis gel of murine hybridoma supernatant from MCT unit: polyacrylamide gel analysis of a mouse monoclonal antibody produced in MCT system. Analysis was performed using standard Laemmli PAGE, 3% stacking gel, 8.7% running gel. Samples in lanes 1, 7, 8, 9 were treated with B-mercaptoethanol (BME). Samples in lanes 3, 4, 5 were treated with iodoacetamide (IAM) to prevent dissociation of antibody molecule. Lane 1, Pharmacia low-molecular-weight standards + BME. Phosphorylase b, m.w. 94K; bovine serum albumin, m.w. 67K; ovalbumin, m.w. 43K. Lane 2, blank. Lane 3, murine antibody purified standard treated with iodoacetamide. Sample deliberately overloaded to bring up impurities. Lane 4, defined low-protein medium concentrate (63-fold). Lane 5, monoclonal antibody eluate from an MCT unit concentrated 55-fold. Lane 6, blank. Lane 7, same as 3 but treated with BME. Lane 8, same as 4 but treated with BME. Lane 9, same as 5 but treated with BME.

be required, depending to some extent on the contaminants present. Low-pressure hydroxyapatite chromatography has been in our experience useful in further purifying final products and simultaneously lowering DNA levels. Formulation of the antibody also depends on the end use and the known antibody stability characteristics.

IV. PRODUCTION OF HUMAN MONOCLONAL ANTIBODIES

Progress in the development of human antibodies as diagnostic or therapeutic reagents, for example in the management of cancer, has been hampered by difficulties in producing significant quantities for even preclinical studies. Preliminary experiments at Bio-Response with the mass culture of human-human hybridomas and Epstein-Barr-virus- (EBV) transformed human B cells suggest that long-term continuous culture systems may be the most effective way to provide human monoclonal antibodies for extensive research and clinical trials.

A. Special Considerations

The production of human monoclonal antibodies is a problem today because most available cell lines secrete human immunoglobulins at very low levels, often around 1 μg/ml/10^6 cells/day or less in conventional static culture. Low secretion rates from cell lines appear to be a universal problem whether those lines are human–human hybridomas, human–mouse hybridomas (or other heteromyelomas), virus-transformed cell lines (e.g., EBV-transformed human B cells), or transfected murine cell lines secreting chimeric immuno-globulins. At this time, there are few prospects on the horizon for better human fusion partner cell lines that would yield hybridomas secreting at levels comparable to productive murine hybridomas.

Another problem is that it is not practical for research groups to generate antibody material for preliminary experiments by trying to grow human ascites tumors in thymectomized or nude mice. The low yields of antibody, the contaminating mouse proteins, the possibility of adventitious agents, and the difficulties in obtaining productive ascites tumors from immunodeficient animals make the bulk production of human antibody by this approach unrealistic. Therefore, in vitro mass culture, particularly if it involves con-tinuous perfusion techniques, is the most plausible means of making human antibodies available for extensive research, let alone for widespread clinical applications.

B. MCT Pilot Studies with Human–Human Hybridomas

Bio-Response has been engaged in a collaborative research effort with the University of California San Diego Cancer Center to produce monoclonal antibodies from human–human hybridomas grown in the MCT continuous perfusion cell culture system. The antibodies bind with high affinity and specificity to glycoprotein antigens found on the cell surfaces of at least five human solid tumors (14). The hybridoma lines were established from human B lymphocytes taken from the regional draining lymph node of a patient with carcinoma of the vulva. These B cells, sensitized to the patient's own tumor, were fused with the 6-thioguanine-resistant human cell line, UC 729-6, developed by Glassy et al. (15). The fusion resulted in stable pseudotetra-ploid human–human hybridomas that secrete IgG for greater than 9 months in continuous conventional culture. Adaptation of these cells to growth in serum-free defined media at Bio-Response enhanced the very low secretion rates about three to five times, up to 1 μg IgG/ml/10^6 cells/day (16,17).

One of these hybridomas, the VLN 3G2.1 line, was cultured in a 1 L hollow fiber ($\sim$300 ml extracapillary volume) MCT unit for nearly 2 months. This line secretes a human IgG3 antibody that binds to a 68,000 MW cell surface glycoprotein bound on several human cell lines (18). The cells were adapted to growth in a commercially available defined medium HL-1 (Ventrex Laboratories, Portland, ME). The static secretion rate in defined medium stabilized at about 1 μg IgG/ml/10^6 cells/day and the cell doubling time

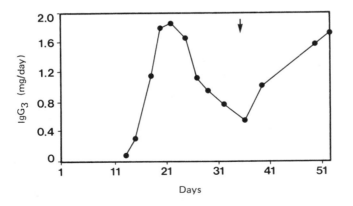

Figure 4 Monoclonal antibody production from a human–human hybridoma: continuous perfusion culture in HL-1 defined medium for production of 25 mg of human IgG3 from 300 ml hollow fiber MCT unit. Arrow indicates cell drain.

remained around 24 hr. Although cell densities exceeded 2×10^7 cells/ml in the MCT unit, antibody production levels ranged from only 0.5 to 3 mg/day as seen in Figure 4. When antibody harvest levels dropped, a cell drain (arrow on Fig. 4) restored the productivity and indicated that maintaining these cells in a log phase growth cycle was more productive than striving to maintain the cells in a stable, low-growth phase. Over a period of 20 days, 25 mg human monoclonal antibody was harvested from this unit, but this material was very dilute on account of the low secretion rate. The antibody was concentrated and sent to Dr. Glassy at the Cancer Center for purification. The antibody has since been biotinylated for conclusive immunohistochemistry studies on frozen sections of human tumors and radiolabeled for preliminary clearance studies in mice.

V. CONCLUSIONS AND FUTURE PERSPECTIVES

The MCT continuous perfusion cell culture system has proven to be a reliable and cost-effective means of producing large quantities of murine monoclonal antibodies at high initial purities. Collectively, over 500 g antibody (IgG, IgM) have been produced at Bio-Response from 18 different murine, rat, and human hybridomas, although antibody contracts represent less than half of the cell culture business at the company. It is quite apparent that the perfusion technology will provide a viable means to address the expected markets for monoclonal antibodies. The success at Bio-Response follows the general trend of the industry in moving towards continuous perfusion culture, emphasizing low-protein defined media, high cell densities, and longer production runs for efficient scale-up.

The long-term, continuous culture of cell lines secreting human monoclonal antibodies will offer the opportunity to produce sufficient material to carry out more extensive research on their potential diagnostic and therapeutic applications. By spreading the initial investment of labor and equipment over a period of months, the gradual accumulation of human antibody material becomes more cost-effective. However, future therapeutic applications of human antibodies, requiring perhaps hundreds of grams of immunoglobulin or more, will depend on the availability of better human fusion partners or genetically engineered cells that secrete antibodies at levels comparable to today's murine hybridomas.

ACKNOWLEDGMENTS

The author acknowledges the cooperation of Dr. Peter Brown, Dr. Maureen Costello, and Barbara Harkonen of Bio-Response and Dr. Mark C. Glassy of

University of California San Diego Cancer Center in the preparation of the manuscript.

REFERENCES

1. Fazekas de St. Groth, S. (1983). Automated production of monoclonal antibodies in A cytostat. *J. Immunol. Methods 56*: 121–136.
2. Jarvis, A. P., Jr. and Grdina, T. A. (1983). Production of biologicals from microencapsulated living cells. *Bio-techniques 1*: 22–27.
3. Littlefield, S. G., Gilligan, K. J., and Larvis, A. P. (1984). Growth and monoclonal antibody production from rat X mouse hybridomas: A comparison of microcapsule culture with conventional suspension culture. *Hybridoma 3*: 75.
4. Birch, J. R., Thompson, P. W., and Boraston, R. (1985). The production of monoclonal antibodies in large-scale cell culture. *Trans. Biochem. Soc. 13*: 10–12.
5. Birch, J. R., Boraston, R., and Wood, L. (1985). Bulk production of monoclonal antibodies in fermenters. *Trends Biotechnol. 3*: 162–166.
6. Seaver, S. S. and Gabriels, J. E. (1985). A membrane-based perfusion system for the continuous production of monoclonal antibody in culture. *Hybridoma 4*: 64.
7. Putnam, J. E., Wyatt, D. E., Pugh, G. G., Noll, L. A., and Lydersen, B. K. (1985). Maximizing antibody production using the Opticell culture system. *Hybridoma 4*: 63.
8. Sinacore, M. S., Geyer, S., Lynch, M., Frye, M., Dobbels, S., and Buehler, R. (1985). Mass culture of hybridoma cells by gel entrapment. *Hybridoma 4*: 64.
9. Knazek, R. A., Gullino, P. M., Kohler, P. O., and Dedrick, R. L. (1972). Cell culture on artificial capillaries: An approach to tissue culture in vitro. *Science 178*: 65.
10. Kopkinson, J. (1985). Hollow fiber cell culture systems for economical cell-product manufacturing. *Bio/Technol. 3*: 225–230.
11. Wiemann, M. C., Ball, E. D., Fanger, M. W., Dexter, D. L., McIntyre, O. R., Bernier, G., Jr., and Calabresi, P. (1983). Human and murine hybridomas: Growth and monoclonal antibody production in the artificial capillary system (abstract). *Clin. Res. 31* (2): 511A.
12. Altshuler, G. L., Dziewulski, D. M., Sowek, J. A., and Belfort, G. (1986). Continuous hybridoma growth and monoclonal antibody production in hollow fiber reactor/separators. *Biotechnol Bioeng. 28*: 646–658.
13. von Wedel, R. J., Mighetto, P. I., Brooks, J., and Juarez-Salinas, H. (1985). Mass culture of hybridomas: Production, purification and characterization of mouse monoclonal AE-1 antibody. *Hybridoma* (Abstracts) *4* (2): 189.
14. Glassy, M. C., Gaffar, S. A., Peters, R. E., and Royston, I. (1985). Human monoclonal antibodies to human cancer cells. In *Monoclonal Antibodies and Cancer Therapy*, UCLA Symposia on Molecular and Cellular Biology,

New Series, Edited by R. A. Reisfeld and S. Sell. New York, Alan R. Liss, *27*: 97.

15. Glassy, M. C., Handley, H. H., Hagiwara, H., and Royston, I. (1983). UC 729-6, a human lymphoblastoid B cell line useful for generating antibody secreting human–human hybridomas. *Proc. Natl. Acad. Sci. USA 80*: 6327–6332.

16. von Wedel, R. J., Glassy, M. C., Mighetto, P. I., and Oakley, R. V. (1985). The mass culture of human–human hybridomas secreting antibodies directed against several human solid tumors. Tissue Culture Association Annual Meeting, June 2–6, 1985.

17. Glassy, M. C., Peters, R. E., and Mikhalez, A. (1987). Growth of human–human hybridomas in serum-free media enhances antibody secretion. *In Vitro*, in press.

18. Glassy, M. C. (1987). Immortalization of human lymphocytes from a tumor involved lymph node. *Cancer Res.*, in press.

19. Laemmli, V. (1970). Cleavage of structural proteins during the assembly of the head of bacterophage T4. *Nature 227*: 680–685.

10

Optimization Techniques for the Production of Monoclonal Antibodies Utilizing Hollow-Fiber Technology

BRADLEY G. ANDERSEN and MICHEAL L. GRUENBERG
Endotronics, Inc., Coon Rapids, Minnesota

I. INTRODUCTION

Hollow-fiber technology has many advantages for large-scale mammalian cell culture:

1. High cell densities ($>10^8$ cells/ml).
2. Efficient distribution of nutrients and removal of metabolic waste products.
3. Secreted proteins can be harvested in a concentrated form, because they cannot pass through 6–10,000 MW cut-off fibers.
4. Cells are immobilized in the fiber bundle, allowing cell-free harvests.
5. Secreted proteins can be harvested in very pure form (60–95%).
6. Hollow-fiber technology is well suited for long-term continuous culture.

Even though these advantages have been well documented for some time (1–8), hollow-fiber technology has not been utilized commercially on a large scale until recently. This is because of the technical problems associated with the scale-up of this technology, some of which are:

1. The need for sophisticated control of the culture environment surrounding the densely packed cells

175

2. The formation of metabolite and oxygen gradients in the hollow fiber bioreactor
3. The lack of sufficient nutrient diffusability through a dense cell mass

These limitations and the solutions we have used to meet them are explained in the following sections.

II. ACUSYST-P SYSTEM

The Acusyst-P cell culture system is designed to automate the production of mammalian cell-secreted products. The system provides controlled conditions for scale-up cell culture through incorporation of advanced hollow-fiber technology, continual media feed, and state-of-the-art process control strategies. The Acusyst-P allows monitoring and feedback control of vital parameters to maintain cell growth, viability, and secretion.

The Acusyst-P consists of two independently controlled flowpaths, which contain 6 hollow fiber cartridges each, or a total of 12 cartridges per instrument (Figure 1). Each hollow-fiber cartridge in the Acusyst-P flowpath has a total fiber surface area of 1.4 cm^2 and a nominal molecular weight cutoff of 6,000–10,000. Cultures within these cartridges routinely reach densities of 5×10^8–10^9 cell/ml. Hence, each instrument can support 10^{11}–10^{12} viable cells over an extended period of time (months).

Process control in the Acusyst-P is specifically designed to meet the requirements of a dense culture. The software uses computer-controlled algorithms to balance nutrient feed, waste removal, and maintain pH at specified setpoints. Critical parameters such as pH, oxygen, glucose, lactic acid, and serum levels fluctuate rapidly in a dense culture, thus a process control technique that responds rapidly is essential. This control strategy relies on continued media feed, online pH, and dissolved oxygen monitoring, and offline glucose and lactic acid monitoring. This strategy, combined with data entry, provides specific control over culture conditions.

In addition to control parameters, the Acusyst-P is capable of continual product harvest, which helps the user to predict future product concentrations. This is especially relevant with cells that are sensitive to product feedback inhibition. In addition to continual product harvest, each flowpath can be gradually weaned from serum, such that dense cultures become essentially serum free. Hollow-fiber cartridge technology provides a demonstrated advantage in this regard, which significantly reduces downstream product purification costs.

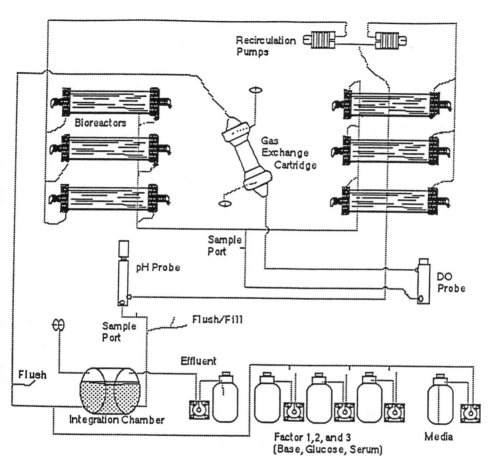

(a)

Figure 1 (a) Acusyst-P flowpath recirculation circuit. Medium is circulated through the lumen of a bank of six hollow-fiber cartridges, 6000–10,000 nominal MW cutoff. The Acusyst-P can support two banks of six cartridges. Cells are on the extracapillary side of the hollow fibers. Circulating medium also flows through a DO probe (where oxygen levels are checked), the gas equilibration cartridge, an integration chamber, and the pH probe. Fresh medium, glucose factor, serum, or base can each be pumped into the system independently via the integration chamber. An equal volume of spent medium is removed from the system at the integration chamber.

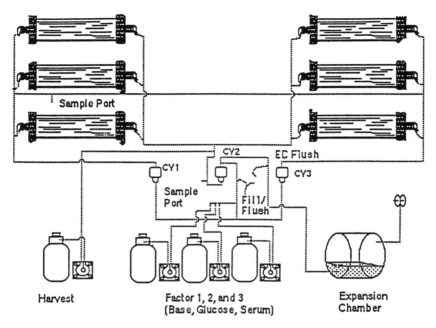

(b)

Figure 1   (Continued)

(b) Extracapillary space flowpath and expansion circuit. The extracapillary space (ECS) of the hollow fiber units contains the hybridoma cells. The ECS are all interconnected and also connected to an expansion chamber. The level of the medium in the expansion chamber is automatically and periodically increased and decreased using a series of check valves (CV 1–3) and pressure differentials. This maintains an even distribution of nutrients and cells in the ECS. Antibody is harvested from the ECS. Base, glucose, serum, or medium can be added to the ECS independently.

III. CONTROL OF THE CULTURE ENVIRONMENT

The need for an advanced system of process control for the extracellular environment is an inherent difficulty with all dense culture scale-up technologies. Systems operating at high cell densities (5×10^8 cells/ml) experience more rapid rates of change in culture conditions than low-density culture (5×10^6 cells/ml) (9,10). The principal reason for this rate of change is that the densely packed cells are exposed proportionally to a smaller volume of media at any one time; thus the buffering and nutrient capacity of the culture media is extremely limited. This causes the loss of sufficient pH control and the rapid accumulation or depletion of metabolites. To overcome these difficulties in hollow-fiber technology, we have developed sophisticated process control software for pH, glucose, and lactate to maintain user-determined setpoints. pH is controlled primarily by gassing, with base addition and medium dilution providing secondary and tertiary control systems. Glucose is controlled by glucose factor addition, with medium addition available as a secondary glucose control capability. Lactate is controlled by base addition and medium dilution.

A. pH Control

The software utilizes a hierarchy of three different algorithms to control pH within ±0.03 pH units. The first algorithm controls the CO_2 mixture. Bicarbonate-buffered culture medium allows pH to be controlled at a setpoint by automatically increasing or decreasing the amount of CO_2 delivered to the gas exchange cartridge (Fig. 1). The second algorithm is base (NaOH) addition to the culture medium, which rejuvenates the buffering capacity of the medium and counters the increased lactic acid production rate of a growing culture. The third control algorithm is medium dilution; this is the most expensive method. Increased medium delivery to the culture effectively increases pH by removing waste products (i.e., lactic acid) more rapidly.

B. Glucose and Lactic Acid Control Strategies

The metabolic data are measured offline and then entered into the computer. The software then calculates medium and glucose pump rate corrections from the entered data based on desired setpoints 24 hr later. The software does this by determining the time in hours between samples, the total volumes pumped by each pump, and the average flowrates of each substance over the sample interval. This information, combined with the known glucose concentrations in medium, glucose factor, and serum (data supplied by the user), provides all information necessary for calculation of glucose comsumption and lactate production values, and for control of pump speeds to maintain the user desired setpoints.

The following definitions will be used in the uptake and production formulas that follow:

Fm = flowrate of medium being added
Fg = flowrate of glucose factor being added
Fs = flowrate of serum factor being added
Fb = flowrate of base addition factor (concentrated NaOH) being added
Gm = concentration of glucose in medium
Gg = concentration of glucose in glucose factor
Gs = concentration of glucose in serum factor
Ft = total flowrate = Fm + Fg + Fs + Fb
E = exp(−FtT/V)
T = time in hours since last sample
V = system volume in milliliters = 1146 + [(190) × (number of cartridges)]

An equal volume of spent medium is removed as fresh medium or other factors are added.

1. Glucose Uptake

Glucose concentration is controlled at a user-defined setpoint by combining medium with a supplemental glucose factor feed. The software first calculates the lactate production rate (LPR) and then the glucose uptake rate (GUR), based on actual sample concentration. The amount of glucose required to maintain a specific level is determined and compared to the glucose contributed through continued media feed. If a need for additional glucose exists, a flow rate is calculated for a supplemental glucose factor feed. Glucose factor feed is accomplished by attaching a separate media source supplemented with 3000 mg% (mg/dl) glucose.

Glucose uptake for the most recent sample period is based on the following formula:

$$GUR = \frac{Gx - FtG - E(Gx - FtGo)}{1 - E}$$

where: G = current glucose reading, Go = previous glucose reading, and Gx = (FmGm) + (FgGg) + (FsGs).

If no fluids have been pumped into the flowpath since the last sample, the uptake rate is defined to be:

$$GUR = \frac{(V)(Go - G)}{T}$$

2. Lactate Production Rate

Similarly to glucose, lactate concentrations are measured offline and data subsequently entered into the computer. The software then calculates the production rate and determines a medium pump rate that controls lactic acid concentration around a predetermined setpoint.

The calculation of lactate production is:

$$LPR = \frac{(Ft)\ (L - LoE)}{1 - E}$$

where Lo = lactate concentration of previous sample and L = lactate concentration of current sample.

If no fluids have been pumped into the flowpath since the last sample, the LPR is defined as

$$LPR = \frac{(V)\ (Lo - L)}{T}$$

3. Glucose and Lactic Acid Projection Formulas

Based on glucose uptake and lactic acid production rates, the software attempts to maintain glucose concentration at the glucose setpoint in each flowpath, and the lactate concentration at the lactate setpoint. The projection is attempted for the 24 hr immediately succeeding the sample; the metabolic calculation algorithm is executed every time sample data are entered, so pump speed estimates are assumed to be constant over the following 24 hr period.

The glucose and lactate levels for any sample period may be determined by rearranging the formulas in the preceding sections.

At time t (defined to be 24 hr after the current sample), the glucose concentration at time t (Gt) and lactate concentration (Lt) will be:

$$Gt = \frac{Gx - GUR + (E)\ (GUR + FtG + Gx)}{Ft}$$

where G = current glucose concentration; and

$$Lt = \frac{(E)\ (FtL - LPR) + LPR}{Ft}$$

where Lt = lactate concentration at time t and L = current lactate concentration.

Optimally, Gt and Lt correspond closely with the user's glucose and lactate setpoints. Direct solution of the projection equation is not possible. The technique used to solve for the necessary pump rate that will give a glucose or lactate concentration acceptably close to the setpoint is a binary search with all variables held constant except flowrate.

The medium pump rate required to control lactate concentration is calculated first, followed by glucose factor rate (using the updated medium pump rate previously calculated), followed by another medium pump adjustment to supplement glucose if the glucose factor pump is unable to satisfy demand. The total volume in the system remains constant since a volume of spent medium equal to that added is simultaneously removed from the system.

IV. CONTROL OF METABOLITE AND OXYGEN GRADIENTS

An additional limitation to scale-up utilizing hollow fibers for the growth of mammalian cells has been the formation of oxygen and metabolite gradients caused by what is referred to as the Starling effect (7,9–13). This is a convective flow through the extracapillary space (ECS) of the cartridge caused by pressure differences from one end of the cartridge to the other in response to lumenal media flow (11 for review). These gradients permit only part of the cell mass within the bioreactor to be at the optimal conditions for growth, while the cells at the outlet of the bioreactor are subjected to depleted media conditions. To resolve this problem, a secondary flow through the ECS of the cartridge is created by controlling the ultrafiltrative flow from the lumen of the fibers past the cell mass. This medium is then automatically transferred into and out of an expansion chamber attached to the ECS of the bioreactor (Fig. 1b). By this method the fluid dynamics of the ECS environment are greatly improved, causing the cells to be bathed with an even distribution of nutrients and improving the removal of waste and inhibitory products (13).

Control of the dissolved oxygen concentration has been found to be extremely important for cell growth and monoclonal antibody production for a variety of hybridomas (10,14). The control of dissolved oxygen and the associated oxygen gradients within the cell mass has been considered one of the missing factors in the use of hollow-fiber technology (10,12). The extent of the oxygen gradients in hollow-fiber bioreactors has recently been thoroughly characterized, and was found to be controlled in this system by variable media delivery rates through the lumen of the hollow fibers (15). Removing the requirement of adding pure oxygen to the gassing mixture eliminates the possibility of oxygen becoming a cytotoxic factor. The next area of interest for the optimization of hollow fiber type systems, along with any other scale-up system, is the effect of nutrient and waste metabolite concentrations on the ability of the cells to grow and, more importantly, to produce.

V. MONOCLONAL ANTIBODY PRODUCTION

A major problem in the large-scale production of monoclonal antibodies in an Acusyst-P has been to determine the most favorable environment for the cells. Our initial approach was to analyze kinetic data from a 5–7-day batch culture. Between 0.5 and 1.0×10^5 cells/ml were inoculated into T25 flasks. Aliquots were removed daily and assayed for glucose, lactate, cell number, pH, and product concentration. A computer program was written that generated curves to fit the kinetic culture. These curves were used to determine the growth rates and production rates per cell number for each hour of the study. A typical hybridoma cell "fingerprint" from this computer model is shown in Figure 2. Cells grown in this manner follow a predictable pattern of an initial lag phase, exponential growth phase, slowing to a preliminary stationary phase, stationary phase, and a subsequent death phase. Glucose consumption follows an initial lag phase, followed by an exponential phase concomitant with the cell growth phase. Lactate is produced in approximately a 1:1 ratio to glucose consumption. pH begins in the range of 7.35–7.45 and decreases steadily with time. Late in the death phase pH may show a slight increase. Product accumulates proportionally to cell growth, but continues to increase even during the death phase. The increase in product concentration during the death phase is associated with increased production per cell, not with intracellular product released from lysed cells (unpublished data). The environmental conditions that cause the shift from stationary phase to death phase is commonly attributed to one or a combination of the following: low nutrient levels, high metabolic waste products, low pH levels, or cellular-produced feedback inhibition (10,14,16). The exact mechanism causing cell population to shift into the death phase is probably an intricate combination of all these factors, and perhaps involves other as yet undefined factors. The essential amino acid concentrations were also tested to determine if their uptake rates followed the trend of the glucose uptake rate. The amino acid uptake rates appeared to follow the glucose uptake rate and it was surprising that, tyrosine, methionine, valine, and lysine were actually utilized very quickly along with L-glutamine for the AFP-27 murine hybridomas tested here (Table 1) (17).

Our initial process control strategy for hybridoma cells was to control the cellular environment so that conditions were not allowed to deteriorate past the environmental conditions associated with the stationary phase. Setpoints

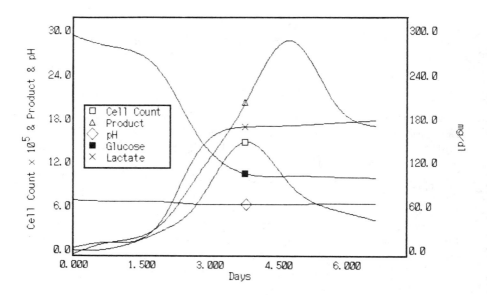

Figure 2 "Fingerprint" of kinetic data of a murine hybridoma AFP-27 producing an IgG.

for pH, glucose, and lactate were selected at the apex of the growth curve (Fig. 3). This process control strategy resulted in very unpredictable production. Table 2 shows production data from four different hybridoma cell lines in an Acusyst-P. Total production ranged from 0.40 to 2.10 g/day (17). No correlation existed between production in a T-flask and production in an Acusyst-P. Another problem was that the production data was not always repeatable from each production run. With the same process control setpoints, production from the same cell line could vary up to 400%. To determine the cause of this variability, we investigated the metabolic kinetic data from two production runs from the same murine hybridoma that resulted in significantly different production.

In the first production run, glucose was consumed and lactate produced until the levels reached the set control points, 150 mg% and 100 mg%, respectively. From that point, glucose and lactate were kept in control. The pH was maintained throughout at 7.15. Total production over a 12 day period was 2.6 g/IgG.

In the second production run, glucose was kept at relatively high levels initially (200 mg%) and then allowed to fall to relatively low levels (125 mg%).

Table 1 Amino Acid Data (μM) for AFP-27 Cells Grown in McCoy's 5A Medium

Days	Cell/ml (× 10⁵)	ARG	LYS	GLN	THR	ALA	VAL	ILE	MET	HIS	GLU	TYR
0	1.17	91	43	905	28	76	37	56	17	56	69	18
1	2.33	96	30	786	11	95	32	47	14	33	66	14
2	9.11	76	19	438	11	101	16	25	6	34	67	5
3	22.2	48	7	331	6	163	9	22	4	31	51	0
4	3.78	46	6	262	6	214	10	20	3	29	29	0

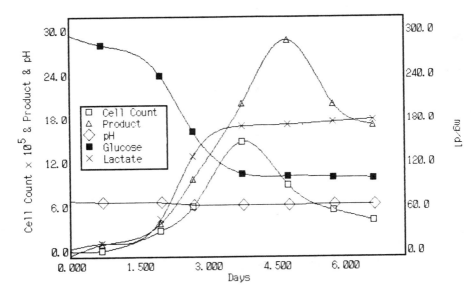

Figure 3 Common "fingerprint" of kinetic data for batch culture with standard operating procedure control parameters selected for murine hybridoma AFP-27.

Lactate was kept low initially (100 mg%) then gradually reached very high levels (200 mg%). The pH gradually fell in time, then rose slightly toward the end of the run. Total production over a 12 day period was 18.55 g/IgG.

These results indicated that the metabolic environment around the cells can have a significant influence on the cellular behavior. Conditions that

Table 2 Hybridoma Production Data from an Acusyst-P

Cell type	Product	Harvest concentration (μg/ml)	Total (g/day)
Mouse X mouse	IgA	5800	1.67
Human X mouse	IgM	420	0.40
Mouse X mouse	IgG	1000	0.50
Human X mouse	IgG2a	1109	2.10

more closely simulated the dynamic environment found in static culture resulted in higher antibody production than the more well controlled environment in the first production run.

This led us to investigate whether we could create separate conditions that would favor cell proliferation or antibody production. The metabolic "fingerprint" for these cells was reexamined to determine growth (cellular proliferation) setpoints. The point on the growth curve where the rate of the increase in cell number was greatest was determined. Glucose and lactate setpoints were determined at that point (see Fig. 4). The pH at this point was very low (about 6.8). This was considered to be too low to initiate cell growth. Therefore, the pH setpoint was selected at the point where the rate of cell division was greatest (see Fig. 4).

Antibody production setpoints were selected at the point where production per cell was greatest (see Fig. 5). Greatest production per cell occurred well into the death phase. Nutrient uptake on a per cell basis, usually characterized by glucose and glutamine utilization, is generally greatest during the exponential growth phase, when the cells are producing the greatest biomass and increasing cell size (10). This uptake rate is commonly between 1.5 and 2.0×10^3 mg/10^5 cell hour, and then slows to nearly zero. An uptake rate of $0.7-1.9 \times 10^4$ mg/10^5 cell hour is commonly seen for glucose by the hybridomas in our laboratory and remains fairly steady during the stationary and death phases. This implies that if the environmental conditions surrounding these latter phases of the growth curve could be maintained, without cell death, the amount of antibody produced per unit of media used would be optimal. We tested the effect of high levels of lactate on cells in static culture (see Fig. 6). Lactate inhibited the growth of cells but did not affect viability. However, high levels of lactate also caused an increase in the production per cell (see Fig. 7) (17). These results were ideal for continuous hollow-fiber culture, since they implied that a confluent culture could be inhibited from growing by high lactate levels allowing the culture to last a longer time. Additionally, the culture would potentially produce more antibody per cell. Therefore, the lactate and glucose production setpoints were selected at the point of highest antibody production per cell. The pH setpoint was selected at the apex of the growth curve (Fig. 5). It has been noted in our laboratory that if the lactate levels in the bioreactors are allowed to reach concentrations above 400 mg%, and pH is not controlled above 6.5, the cells die almost immediately. However, under the same conditions if the pH is controlled at 6.8 or above, there are no detrimental effects on the cells (unpublished data).

The comparison of growth phase parameters to production phase parameters gave the results expected. The metabolic growth parameters, GUR and LPR, showed that the flowpaths controlled at the growth phase conditions

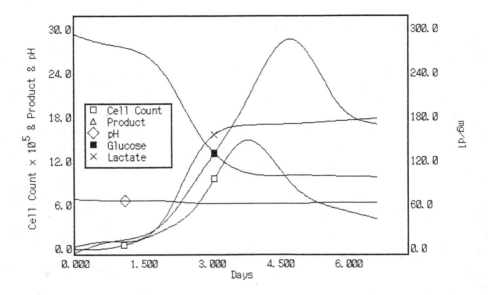

Figure 4   Growth phase parameters selected for AFP-27 murine hybridoma.

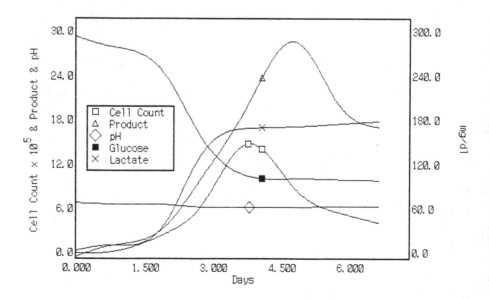

Figure 5   Production phase parameters selected for AFP-27 murine hybridoma.

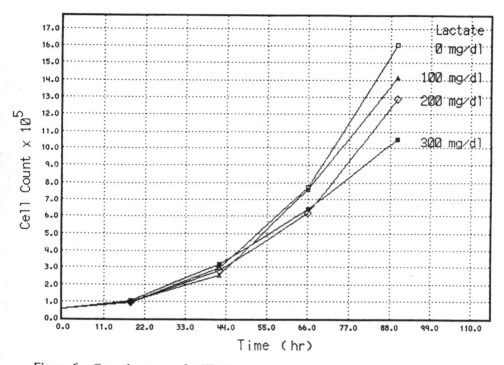

Figure 6   Growth curves of AFP-27 hybridoma cells grown in varying lactate concentrations.

increased their metabolic rates exponentially (Fig. 8). Since these metabolic rates are primarily dependent on the viable cell number, one may assume that the cell population is increasing at a similar rate. The calculated doubling time of the cells in the system utilizing this metabolic data, was about 22 hr, compared to 18 hours in batch culture systems.

The systems controlled at the production phase conditions showed the opposite response compared to the growth phase systems. When the flow-paths were controlled at the production phase parameters, the cells repeatedly did not show any substantial increase in their metabolic rates (Fig. 8), implying a near constant viable cell population of 2×10^9 cells, based on metabolic rates. One may speculate that metabolic rates do not increase in this system because the death rate is equal to the growth rate within the cell population. If this were true, the visible cell density should have increased as the concentration of dead cells increased. However, there was no substantial increase in

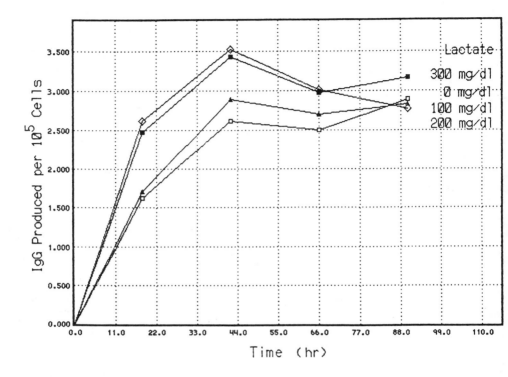

Figure 7 Production of IgG per cell number for AFP-27 hybridoma cells grown in varying lactate concentrations.

the visible cell mass during these experimental runs. The differences between the cells grown at the growth phase and production phase parameters can easily be seen in the metabolic rates shown in Figure 8.

With this data on growth and production phase parameters, it was possible to grow the hybridomas to high densities quickly and then shift to new control parameters that would keep the cells at or near a stable population. This approach, in contrast to conventional production systems, would now allow for product to be removed sooner and at a higher concentration. The metabolic rates for this new control strategy compared to the rates at the standard control conditions are shown in Figure 9. These show that during the growth phase there is a substantial increase in the cellular rate of metabolism, and that after the cells had finished proliferating (~ day 18), it was possible to maintain a highly viable culture during the "antibody production" phase. Figure 10 shows the difference in production rates for these two culture

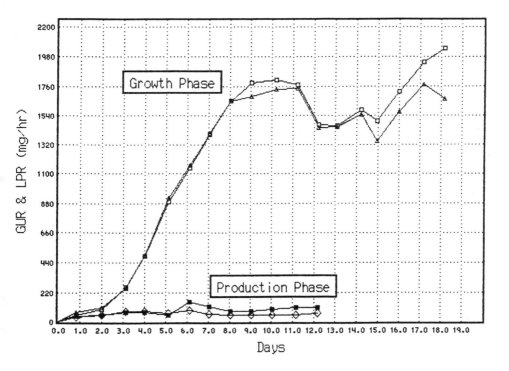

Figure 8   Comparison of glucose uptake rate (GUR) (□, ■) and lactate production rate (LPR) (◊, △) for growth phase and product phase setpoints.

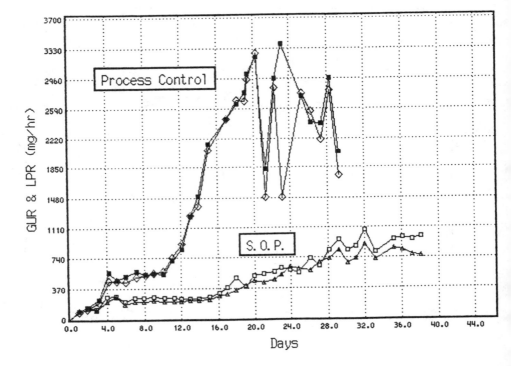

Figure 9   Comparison of glucose uptake rate (GUR) (□, ■) and lactate production rate (LPR) (◊, △) for the standard operating procedure (S.O.P.) and enhanced process control.

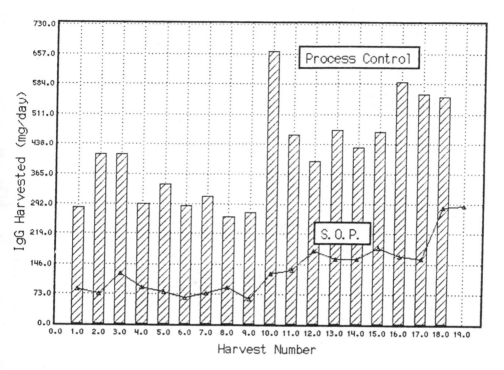

Figure 10   Comparison of production per day of one flowpath in an Acusyst-P between S.O.P. and in the enhanced process control.

strategies. In the culture that was grown quickly and then maintained at antibody production setpoints, there was an increase in production of about 100% over the standard setpoints.

VI. CONCLUSIONS AND DISCUSSION

For the optimization of monoclonal antibody production from hybridomas, a controlled extracellular environment is necessary. Utilizing this control in hollow fiber systems allows optimal cell growth in vitro with the ability for subsequent inhibition of growth and maintenance of a viable cell population for antibody production. The preliminary data shown here imply that selecting the environmental parameters associated with the cellular response desired will allow that response to be maintained in an "environmentally-controlled" hollow-fiber cartridge. For optimal production of monoclonal antibodies from hybridomas utilizing hollow fiber technology, it is necessary to use two sets of control parameters, one for cell growth and another for antibody/ product production. This strategy allows for the achievement of high cell viability in dense culture for maximum antibody production. Furthermore, this strategy could become a standardized method to determine process control strategies for any cell line.

REFERENCES

1. Knazek, R. A., Gullino, P. M., Koher, P. O., and Dedric, R. L. (1972). Cell culture on artificial capillaries: An approach to tissue growth in-vitro. *Science 178*: 65–67.
2. Knazek, R. A., Kohler, P. O., and Gullino, P. M. (1974). Hormone production by cells grown in-vitro on artificial capillaries. *Exp. Cell Res. 84*: 251–254.
3. Knazek, R. A. (1974). Solid tissue masses formed in-vitro form cells cultured on artificial capillaries. *Fed. Proc. 33*: 1978–1981.
4. Ratner, P. L., Cleary, M. L., and Jones, E. (1978). Production of "rapid-harvest" Moloney murine leukemia virus by continuous cell culture on synthetic capillaries. *J. Virol. 26*: 536–539.
5. David, G. S., Reisfeld, R. A., and Chino, T. H. (1978). Continuous production of carcinoembryonic antigen in hollow fiber cell culture units: Brief communication. *J. Natl. Cancer Inst. 60*: 303–306.
6. Calabresi, P., McCarthy, K. L., Dexter, D. L., Cummings, F. J., and Rotman, B. (1981). Monoclonal antibody production in artificial capillary cultures. *Proc. Am. Assoc. Cancer Res. 22*: 302.
7. Ehrlich, K. C., Stewart, E., and Klein, E. (1978). Artificial capillary perfusion cell culture: Metabolic studies. *In Vitro 14*: 443–450.
8. Ku, K., Kuo, M. J., Delente, J., Wildi, B. S., and Feder, J. (1981). Development of a hollow-fiber system for large-scale culture of mammalian cells. *Biotechnol. Bioeng. 23*: 79–95.
9. Altshuler, G. L., Dziewulski, D. M., Sowek, J. A., and Belfort, G. (1986). Continuous hybridoma growth and monoclonal antibody production in hollow fiber reactors/separators. *Biotechnol. Bioeng. 28*: 646–658.
10. Spier, R. E. (1986). The large-scale production of monoclonal antibodies "in vitro". (In press.)
11. Schratter, P. (1976). Cell culture with synthetic capillaries. Amicon Corp.
12. Hu, W.-S. and Wang, D. I. C. (1986). Mammalian cell culture technology: A review from an engineering perspective. In *Mammalian Cell Technology*. Edited by W. G. Thilly. Addison-Wesley.
13. Hirschel, M. (1986). An automated hollow fiber system for the large scale manufacture of mammalian cell secreted products. In *Large Scale Cell Culture Technology*. Edited by B. K. Lydersen. Carl Hanser.

14. Reuveny, S., Velez, D., Macmillan, J. D., and Miller, L. (1986). Factors affecting cell growth and monoclonal antibody production in stirred reactors. *J. Immunol. Methods 86*: 53–59.
15. Tyo, M. (1986). (manuscript in progress).
16. Bettger, W. J. and McKeehan, W. L. (1986). Mechanisms of cellular nutrition. *Physiol. Rev. 66*: 1–35.
17. Ostlie, N., Potter, A., and Sours, D. (1986). Endotronics in-house data.

III

PURIFICATION OF MONOCLONAL ANTIBODIES

11

Affinity Purification of Monoclonal Antibody from Tissue Culture Supernatant Using Protein A-Sepharose CL-4B

SHWU-MAAN LEE*
Program Resources, Inc., National Cancer Institute–Frederick Cancer Research Facility, National Institutes of Health, Frederick, Maryland

I. INTRODUCTION

Protein A is a protein with a molecular weight of 42,000, isolated from the cell wall of *Staphylococcus aureus* (1). Its ability to interact with immunoglobulin (Ig), mainly IgG, from mammalian species has been demonstrated (2). Subsequent studies (3,4) have indicated that protein A reacts with the Fc structure of IgG. It is believed that the aromatic side chain interactions, a combination of π–π and hydrophobic interactions, are involved (5). The IgG-binding properties of protein A make affinity chromatography with protein A-Sepharose CL-4B an attractive method for purifying monoclonal antibodies. We describe here the large-scale affinity purification of a murine antimelanoma monoclonal antibody, 9.2.27, from tissue culture supernatant and the evaluation of final bulk product. A more detailed description of this topic has been published (6). The production of this antibody in stirred culture has been detailed in Chapter 6 by William B. Lebherz III.

II. METHODS DEVELOPMENT

The isolation of Ig classes and subclasses from various mammalian species using protein A-Sepharose has been thoroughly reviewed (7–9). In the mouse, IgG_{2a}, IgG_{2b}, and IgG_3 bind, whereas IgG_1 and IgM bind weakly if at all (10,11). Binding is highly dependent on pH conditions, with stronger binding

---

Present affiliation: Genex Corporation, Gaithersburg, Maryland.

199

occurring at pH 7.0–8.5 and weaker binding below pH 7.0. The methods most commonly used to elute antibody from protein A-Sepharose involve either a chaotropic ion (11) or solutions of low pH (10). Elution with low pH solution is preferable, because the removal of a chaotropic ion is very time consuming. The highest pH that results in complete elution should be used to preserve antibody activity. Mouse IgG_1 is usually eluted at pH 6–7, IgG_{2a} at pH 4.5–5.0, IgG_{2b} at pH 3.5–4.0, and IgG_3 at pH 4.5 (8,12). Elution methods using the competing ligand Gly-Tyr have been tested, but the yields were poor (5).

The 9.2.27 monoclonal antibody, which has been fully characterized as a murine IgG_{2a}, recognizes a melanoma-associated 250K dalton glycoprotein/proteoglycan (13). The methods development for 9.2.27 monoclonal antibody purification was performed in a 5 or 10 ml (Pharmacia K16, diameter = 1.6 cm) protein A-Sepharose CL-4B (Pharmacia) column. Washing and elution pHs were optimized with buffers of progressively lower pH. For 9.2.27 monoclonal antibody, we found that binding and washing were effective at pH 8.2–8.4, washing at pH 7.0 or 6.0 caused a small leakage of the antibody, and elution at pH 4.5 was a simple and effective method.

The binding capacity of the affinity beads was determined by passing the antibody solution through the column until the antibody appeared in the column effluent. At this point, the column was fully saturated and the amount of antibody eluted indicated the capacity of the gel. For 9.2.27 antibody, the binding capacity is 20–30 mg antibody per gram of freeze-dried protein A-Sepharose CL-4B.

As described in Chapter 6, a typical antibody concentration that can be achieved using large-scale suspension cultures of 9.2.27 hybridoma is usually 60–120 μg/ml. A 500 ml protein A-Sepharose column, which is equivalent to 150 g freeze-dried gel, can bind 3–4.5 g 9.2.27 antibody; thus a large volume of culture supernatant must be processed through a relatively small column bed when suspension culture systems are used for bulk antibody production. To reduce column loading time, culture supernatants were concentrated before loading. This can be accomplished by either ammonium sulfate precipitation following dialysis or by ultrafiltration. The latter method was used, because it is less time consuming and can be easily scaled-up.

A Pellicon (Millipore) ultrafiltration system with polysulfone membranes of 100,000 nominal molecular weight cut off (NMWCO) was used to concentrate 9.2.27 antibody from tissue culture supernatants. The membrane filter area was increased according to the scale of operation. Antibody recovery was essentially quantitative (Table 1). However, the ultrafiltration membrane retained 95% of the total protein; therefore, as judged by specific activity, the purity of the antibody remained the same. The crude protein mixture

Table 1 Concentration of Tissue Culture Supernatant Using Ultrafiltration[a]

	Volume (L)	Antibody concentration[b] (mg/ml)	Protein concentration[c] (mg/ml)	Total antibody[b] (g)	Total protein[c] (g)	Specific activity[d] (mg antibody/ mg protein)
Cell culture supernatant	7.2	0.188	4.62	1.4	33	0.041
Concentrate	0.5	3.20	60.0	1.6	30	0.053
Permeate	7.0	0.002	0.31	0.01	2	0.006

[a]Ultrafiltration was performed with a 5 ft.² polysulfone membrane cassette (100,000 NMWCO; Millipore).
[b]Determined using ELISA.
[c]Determined using Bio-Rad dye binding assay.
[d]Antibody concentration/protein concentration.

was not significantly fractionated, because gel polarization occurred during ultrafiltration which effectively prevented an adequate separation (14).

In Tables 1–3, the antibody concentration was determined using an enzyme-linked immunosorbent assay (ELISA) similar to that described by Abrams et al. (15), and the protein was determined using the Bio-Rad dye binding assay with bovine IgG as a standard (16). Affinity-purified goat antimouse IgG and IgM (Kirkegaard Perry Laboratories, Inc., Gaithersburg, MD) was used as the capture antibody, goat antimouse IgG alkaline phosphatase conjugate (Sigma) was used for color development, and mouse myeloma IgG_{2a} (RPC 5, Litton) was used as a standard. This assay quantitated active mouse IgG_{2a}, and assumed that IgG_{2a} was the only mouse antibody in the monoclonal antibody preparation. However, it is not a specific assay for the 9.2.27 antibody and it does not give information about immunoreactivity.

III. SCALE–UP OF PURIFICATION PROCESS

Once the binding pH, elution pH, and column capacity were established, the procedure was scaled-up by increasing the column diameter to maintain the same linear flow rate in production columns as in laboratory columns (17). Bed volume was determined by the amount of antibody to be produced in each run and by the binding capacity of the gel beads. Routinely, only half of the available capacity of the gel was used to minimize the possibility of overloading, which would result in the leaking of antibody into the column wash and reduce the yield.

Because the column gel media often constituted the major cost of large-scale chromatography, the production-scale column was protected. A pre-column of Sephadex G-25 or Sepharose CL-4B was used to adsorb cell debris from tissue culture supernatant concentrates, thus extending the life of the protein A-Sepharose column. Columns were stored in 0.02% sodium azide to avoid bacterial contamination. When the columns were used in the production of clinical grade antibody under the conditions of good manufacturing practices (GMP), the removal of sodium azide had to be verified before the tissue culture supernatant concentrate was introduced. The ferric chloride method (18) was a simple analysis for residual azide. This method also detected residual thiocyanate used for column regeneration. Appendix 2 outlines the procedure for purifying 9.2.27 monoclonal IgG_{2a} from suspension cell culture supernatants.

Table 2 shows the results of several column runs using the procedure described in Appendix 2. Single-step chromatography resulted in a 60- to 140-fold purification of this antibody. The yield ranged from 50 to 160%. The specific activity of purified antibody ranged from 1 to 3. Theoretically,

Table 2 Purification of 9.2.27 Antibody by Protein A–Sepharose Column Chromatography

Column number	Total antibody applied[a] (g)	Total protein applied (g)	Specific activity of cell culture supernatant concentrate (mg antibody/mg protein)	Total antibody recovered[a] (g)	Total protein recovered (g)	Specific activity of purified antibody (mg antibody/mg protein)	Purification (fold)	Yield (%)
1	4.8	269	0.018	2.2	2.0	1.1	61	46
2	5.8	275	0.021	3.7	2.5	1.4	68	64
3	5.5	275	0.020	3.7	2.2	1.6	82	67
4	5.4	298	0.018	7.7	3.1	2.5	140	140
5	4.1	223	0.018	6.6	2.9	2.2	120	160

[a]Determined using ELISA.

the specific activity of antibody should be 1 or less. The variations in purification factor, yield, and specific activity are conceivably due to the variations in the antibody assay, ELISA. The 10-fold serial dilutions made in the plates are probably the main source of variations.

IV. PRODUCT EVALUATION

Two lots of bulk sterile 9.2.27 monoclonal antibody were manufactured. Lot XX03 contained 11 g antibody, as determined by ELISA and protein assay, and lot F10001 contained 32 g antibody when tested with ELISA and 26 g when tested with the protein assay. Lots XX03 and F10001 were constituted with the antibody pooled from 7 and 16 column runs, respectively. The antibody of lots XX03 and F10001 was produced in two and six batches of suspension cultures (280 L/batch), respectively. The results of final product analysis are summarized in Table 3, including evaluations of protein, mouse antibody, endotoxin, protein A, bovine IgG, and DNA levels, as well as purity, sterility, mycoplasma, reverse transcriptase activity, and specific activity. Each of the analyses will be discussed individually in the following sections.

A. Purity

1. Reducing Gel

A reducing sodium dodecyl sulfate (SDS) polyacrylamide gel of the 9.2.27 monoclonal antibody final product is illustrated in Figure 1. In addition to heavy and light chains, a contaminant protein of 27,000 daltons constituting about 10% of the final product is visible in the gel. Light-chain multiplicity in purified monoclonal antibody preparations has been reported (19). Hydroxyapatite chromatography with gradient elution has been found to resolve the heterogeneous monoclonal antibodies (19,20). However, when the 9.2.27 antibody final product was further subjected to hydroxyapatite column chromatography, an inactive fraction was not found and the immunoreactivity of the antibody was determined (21) to be about 80% (Dr. A. C. Morgan, personal communication). These observations did not support the speculation that the contaminating protein in the gel was an extraneous antibody light chain.

2. Nonreducing Gel

Figure 2 is a nonreducing SDS gel of the final product. Aside from the non-reduced IgG molecule, at least two low-molecular-weight bands (145,000 and 84,000 daltons) are visible. The 145,000 dalton band, which is not detectable in the reducing gel, may be an IgG molecule with some posttranslational modifications (proteolysis, glycosylations, etc.). We have observed a similar

Table 3 9.2.27 Monoclonal Antibody: Final Product Analysis

	Results	
Assays	Lot XX03	Lot F10001
Protein (mg/ml)	19.3	15.6
Mouse antibody[a] (mg/ml)	19.0	19.2
Endotoxin (ng/ml)	15.1	17.5
Protein A (ng/ml)	72.0	<3.9
Bovine IgG (mg/ml)	1.05	0.38
Sterility	Negative	Negative
Mycoplasma	Negative	Negative
Reverse transcriptase activity	Negative	Negative
Specific activity	0.98	1.2
DNA (μg/ml)	2.62	—
SDS gel	>90% pure	>90% pure
Isoelectric point	7.5, 7.3, 7.1, 6.9, 6.8, 6.7, and 6.6	7.5, 7.3, 7.1, 6.8, and 6.7

[a]Determined using ELISA.

band in another purified monoclonal antibody isolated from mouse ascites fluid (Lee et al., unpublished result). Others have also reported that monoclonal antibody light chain does not migrate as a single band in gel electrophoresis (22).

In this gel, the IgG molecule and the 200,000 dalton molecular weight marker migrated the same distance. Instead of being a 150,000 dalton molecule, the nonreduced IgG had an observed molecular weight of 200,000 daltons. There are several possible reasons for this discrepancy. First, the relative mobility of proteins above 100,000 daltons is influenced by loading conditions such as sample conductivity. For this reason, multiple molecular weight standards bracketing the IgG molecule should be included for reliable molecular weight determinations (23). Second, glycoproteins show impaired SDS binding and may yield lowered electrophoretic mobilities (24).

3. Isoelectric Focusing Gel

Figure 3 is an isoelectric focusing gel of the final product. The isoelectric points are listed in Table 3. The charge heterogeneity is probably the

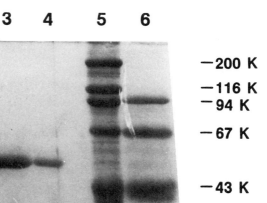

Figure 1   Reducing SDS PAGE (1.5 mm thickness, 10% gel) of affinity-purified 9.2.27 monoclonal antibody. Gels were stained with Coomassie blue. Lanes 1 and 2: 9.2.27 antibody (lot XX03), 6 μg and 1.2 μg, respectively; lanes 3 and 4: 9.2.27 antibody (lot F10001), 6 μg and 1.2 μg, respectively; lane 5: high-molecular-weight protein marker (Bio-Rad); lane 6: low-molecular-weight protein marker (Pharmacia).

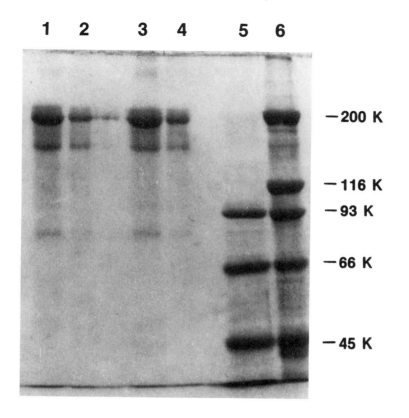

Figure 2 Nonreducing SDS PAGE (6% gel) of 9.2.27 monoclonal antibody. Lanes 1 and 2: 9.2.27 antibody (lot XX03), 6 μg and 1.2 μg, respectively; lanes 3 and 4: 9.2.27 antibody (lot F10001), 6 μg and 1.2 μg, respectively; lane 5: low-molecular-weight protein marker (Pharmacia); lane 6: high-molecular-weight protein marker (Bio-Rad).

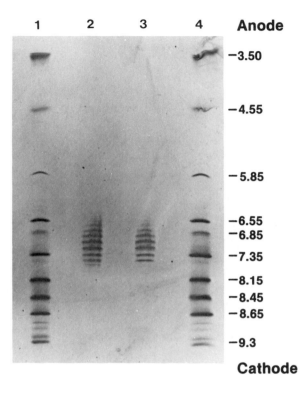

Figure 3 Isoelectric focusing gel of affinity-purified 9.2.27 monoclonal antibody. The focusing was performed on Ampholine PAG plates (LKB, pH range 3.5–9.5). Lanes 1 and 4: isoelectric point calibration mixture (Pharmacia); lane 2: 9.2.27 antibody (lot XX03), 20 μg; lane 3: 9.2.27 antibody (lot F10001), 15 μg.

result of posttranslational modification and variations in the extent of glycosylation (25).

B. Sterility, Mycoplasma, and Specific Activity

From the analysis presented in Table 3, the 9.2.27 final product was sterile and free of mycoplasma contamination. The specific activity (mg mouse antibody as determined by ELISA/mg total protein) of the antibody was 0.98 and 1.2 for lots XX03 and F10001, respectively. The high specific activity indicated that the 9.2.27 antibody was not denatured with acid elution. However, some antibodies are sensitive to acidic pH and have been shown to have reduced activity after low pH elution (26).

C. Viral Activity and Nucleic Acid Level

Monoclonal antibodies are the products of malignant hybridoma cell lines and might contain viruses or nucleic acids that could adversely affect the human recipient. A reverse transcriptase assay (27) was used to determine that the final product had no detectable retrovirus activity. Fluorometric quantitation (28) indicated that lot XX03 contained 2.6 μg/ml DNA against a standard preparation of 9.2.27 DNA. Because false-positive DNA reactions may result from the binding of fluorescent dye with high concentrations of antibody, this method requires further validation.

The acceptable level of DNA in injectable biological products has not been established; however, a maximal upper limit of 1–10 pg DNA per injectable dose has been proposed (29). To detect low levels of DNA, the Food and Drug Administration (FDA) has suggested a hybridization analysis using nick-translated hybridoma cell DNA (30). Because we experienced difficulties with this DNA assay in the presence of milligram quantities of proteins, DNA data for lot F10001 were not available.

D. Protein A Content

Protein A-Sepharose CL-4B consists of staphylococcal protein A covalently coupled to Sepharose CL-4B using the cyanogen bromide method (31). The ligand is monovalently coupled to Sepharose through N-substituted isourea bonds, which are not completely stable (32). These conjugates exhibit a small but constant "leakage" of the ligands from the solid matrix (32,33). Using an ELISA (34), we determined the protein A content of the final product to be 72 and 3.9 ng/ml in lots XX03 and F10001, respectively. Because protein A was detected by this ELISA in all column fractions throughout the loading, washing, and elution stages (34), the leakage was not due to the extreme pH.

The protein A level appeared to be low in the second lot of the product (F10001) purified from the same column. By screening the column fractions throughout the production process, it was observed that the level of protein A leaching decreased with column use (34). This phenomenon indicates that most of the protein A that could leach had been washed off in the first several column runs.

Protein A contamination of the antibody final product may cause side effects in humans. However, there are at present no FDA guidelines for the maximal level of protein A contamination in injectable clinical grade monoclonal antibodies. Protein A affinity adsorbents activated with reagents other than cyanogen bromide are also available. However, the stability of these linkages was not tested.

E. Bovine IgG Level

The culture medium used in the production of the 9.2.27 antibody included 7% fetal bovine serum (M.A. Bioproducts), which contained 0.2 mg/ml bovine IgG according to the manufacturer's specifications. The culture medium thus contained 14 μg/ml bovine IgG. Bovine IgG_{2a} and small amounts of IgG_1 can bind to protein A-Sepharose and are both eluted at an acidic pH (35). Thus, bovine IgG from serum might contaminate monoclonal antibody produced in tissue culture medium containing a serum supplement, especially if the antibody is purified with protein A-Sepharose chromatography. Bovine IgG levels were determined to be 1.05 and 0.38 mg/ml in lots XX03 and F10001, respectively.

The production of antimouse antibodies in response to mouse monoclonal antibody was observed in human clinical trials (36). Bovine IgG contamination may induce similar antibovine antibodies in patients. Underwood et al. (37) suggested removing bovine IgG from bovine serum with protein A-Sepharose before introducing the serum into the culture medium and then purifying the monoclonal antibody on a second protein A-Sepharose column. However, at present time the FDA has no guidelines for acceptable levels of bovine IgG contamination in clinical products.

F. Endotoxin Level

The endotoxin levels of lots XX03 and F10001 were determined to be 15.1 and 17.5 ng/ml, respectively, using the limulus amebocyte lysate (LAL) assay (38). The rabbit pyrogen test (described in 21 Code of Federal Regulations 610.13) indicated that lot F10001 was pyrogenic.

An effort was made to determine sources of endotoxins (Table 4). The endotoxin levels in culture medium were very low (0.018 ng/ml) and usually

Table 4   Endotoxin Levels at Various Stages of 9.2.27 Antibody Production[a]

Steps	Endotoxin[b] (ng/ml)
1. Tissue culture medium before inoculation	0.018
2. Tissue culture medium prior to cell removal	0.039
3. Supernatant of culture medium before Pellicon concentration	8.2
4. Concentrated tissue culture supernatant	172
5. Concentrated culture supernatant after Zeta potential filtration	37
6. Purified antibody from protein A-Sepharose column	0.5–2
7. Concentrated antibody bulk product	17.5

[a]Data kindly provided by William B. Lebherz III, Program Resources, Inc., NCI-FCRF.
[b]Chromogenic LAL assay was used.

reflected the contribution of the raw materials such as fetal bovine serum, water, and others. The terminal endotoxin levels in uncontaminated fermentors were also very low (0.039 ng/ml). During the centrifuging, the culture supernatants were held 24 hr in a chilled tank and the endotoxin levels increased drastically (8.2 ng/ml). Subsequent Pellicon ultrafiltration further concentrated the endotoxins (172 ng/ml). Fortuitously, we achieved a significant reduction of endotoxins (37 ng/ml) when crude antibody concentrate was clarified with 2 μm Zeta potential filters (Pall). The endotoxins were further removed from the column wash. Usually, the levels were as low as 0.05 ng/ml in the final wash fraction through the protein A-Sepharose column, but the levels increased to 0.5–2 ng/ml as the antibody was eluted from the column. Prewashing the column with depyrogenated elution buffer before loading did not reduce the level of endotoxin in the column eluent. These observations indicate that some endotoxin from the culture supernatants may nonspecifically bind to an affinity column or may physically associate with the antibody and thus copurify with the product. Affinity chromatography has been reported to be effective for pyrogen removal (39); however, we found that one-step chromatography has a limited ability to remove endotoxins completely from process streams containing high levels of endotoxins. Column chromatography may significantly reduce the level of endotoxins, but the endotoxin level may be increased if the product must be subsequently concentrated by ultrafiltration. Bacterial endotoxins have been shown to exist as high-molecular-weight aggregates of greater than 10^6 daltons

(40). These aggregates are retained by ultrafiltration membranes and concentrated with the final antibody product.

Various methods have been proposed for endotoxin removal, including charge-modified filters (41,42), affinity chromatography with polymyxin B-Sepharose (43) or with nitrogen-containing heterocyclic compounds as ligands (44), ultrafiltration (45,46), ion-exchange chromatography (47), adsorption (48,49), and density gradient centrifugation (50). However, only a few of these methods are suitable for removing endotoxins from protein products. The removal of endotoxin from protein with gel permeation high performance liquid chromatography (HPLC) in the presence of 0.05% sodium taurocholate (51) seems to be a promising approach, because the detergent can break the association between protein and endotoxin aggregates; however, the detergent must subsequently be removed. A recent report (52) indicates that polymyxin B-Sepharose will bind some but not all endotoxins.

To reduce endotoxins, various postchromatographic treatments were evaluated on neutralized column fractions. Adsorption with aluminum oxide gel caused complete loss of antibody and endotoxin. However, detailed concentration and pH-dependent studies were not pursued. Batch adsorption with Detoxi-gel (Pierce) did not remove any endotoxin. Filtration with Zeta potential filters (Posidyne 2 μm filter, Pall) removed 40% of the residual endotoxins, but 20% of the product was lost as well. Depth filtration with Zeta plus 1 DEP filter (AMF Cuno) resulted in complete loss of the antibody.

V. CONCLUSION

Protein A-Sepharose CL-4B column chromatography is a convenient method for monoclonal antibody purification. The single-step purification procedure could easily be scaled-up to produce gram quantities of monoclonal antibody. In addition, the procedure significantly increased antibody purity and reduced endotoxin contamination. However, only limited purification and endotoxin reduction can be achieved for the weakly bound IgG subclasses. The single-step affinity method does not always purify antibody to homogeneity. The product is generally satisfactory for in vitro studies. However, before the procedure can be used to produce clinical grade material, the problems of protein A leaching, bovine IgG contamination, residual endotoxin levels, minor protein contamination, and possible nucleic acid contamination must be addressed. The FDA has no guidelines for acceptable levels of protein contamination in injectable monoclonal antibodies. An additional ion-exchange chromatography step might remove the minor protein and nucleic acid contaminants and possibly reduce endotoxin levels.

ACKNOWLEDGMENTS

The author acknowledges the valuable comments of Dr. Michael Flickinger and the assistance of her collaborators: Dr. Mark Gustafson, William B. Lebherz III, Dr. A. C. Morgan, Dr. Gary Muschik, Dana Pickle, Penny Hylton, Ralph Hopkins III, Pamela Clark, Joe Zalewski, and Marie Wroble.

This project has been funded at least in part with Federal funds from the Department of Health and Human Services, under contract number N01-CO-23910 with Program Resources, Inc. The contents of this publication do not necessarily reflect the views of the Department of Health and Human Services, nor does mention of trade names, commercial products, or organizations imply endorsement by the U.S. Government.

REFERENCES

1. Sjoquist, J., Movitz, J., Johansson, I.-B., and Hjelm, H. (1972). Localization of protein A in the bacteria. *Eur. J. Biochem. 30*: 190–194.
2. Forsgren, A. and Sjoquist, J. (1966). Protein A from *S. aureus*, pseudo-immune reaction with human γ-globulin. *J. Immunol. 97*: 822–827.
3. Gustafson, G. T., Sjoquist, J., and Stalenheim, G. (1967). Protein A from *Staphylococcus aureus*, Arthus-like reaction produced in rabbits by inter-action of protein A and human γ-globulin. *J. Immunol. 98*: 1178–1181.
4. Gustafson, G. T., Stalenheim, G., Forsgren, A., and Sjoquist, J. (1968). Protein A from *Staphylococcus aureus*, production of anaphylaxis-like cutaneous and systematic reactions in non-immunized guinea pigs. *J. Immunol. 100*: 530–534.
5. Bywater, R., Eriksson, G.-B., and Ottosson, T. (1983). Desorption of immunoglobulins from protein A-Sepharose CL-4B under mild conditions. *J. Immunol. Methods 64*: 1–6.
6. Lee, S.-M., Gustafson, M. E., Pickle, D. J., Flickinger, M. C., Muschik, G. M., and Morgan, A. C. Jr. (1986). Large-scale purification of a murine anti-melanoma monoclonal antibody. *J. Biotechnology 4*: 189–204.
7. Langone, J. J. (1982). Applications of immobilized protein A in immuno-chemical techniques. *J. Immunol. Methods 55*: 277–296.
8. Lindmark, R., Kerstin, T.-T., and Sjoquist, J. (1983). Binding of immuno-globulins to protein A and immunoglobulin levels in mammalian sera. *J. Immunol. Methods 62*: 1–13.
9. Goding, J. W. (1978). Use of staphylococcal protein A as an immuno-logical reagent. *J. Immunol. Methods 20*: 241–253.
10. Ey, P. L., Prowse, S. J., and Jenkin, C. R. (1978). Isolation of pure IgG_1, IgG_{2a}, and IgG_{2b} immunoglobulins from mouse serum using protein A-Sepharose. *Immunochemistry 15*: 429–436.

11. Mackenzie, M. R., Warner, N. L., and Mitchell, G. F. (1978). The binding of murine immunoglobulins to staphylococcal protein A. *J. Immunol. 120*: 1493–1496.
12. Seppala, I., Sarvas, H., Peterfy, F., and Makela, O. (1981). The four subclasses of IgG can be isolated from mouse serum by using protein A-Sepharose. *Scand. J. Immunol. 14*: 335–342.
13. Morgan, A. C. Jr., Galloway, D. R., and Reisfeld, R. A. (1981). Production and characterization of monoclonal antibody to a melanoma specific glycoprotein. *Hybridoma 1*: 27–36.
14. Nelsen, L. L. and Reti, A. R. (1979). Ultrafiltration in plasma fractionation. *Pharm. Technol. 3*: 51–56.
15. Abrams, P. G., Ochs, J. J., Giardina, S. L., Morgan, A. C., Wilburn, S. B., Wilt, A. R., Oldham, R. K., and Foon, K. A. (1984). Production of large quantities of human immunoglobulin in the ascites of athymic mice: Implications for the development of anti-human idiotype monoclonal antibodies. *J. Immunol. 132*: 1611–1613.
16. Bradford, M. (1976). A rapid and sensitive method for quantitation of microgram quantities of protein utilizing the principle of protein-dye binding. *Anal. Biochem. 72*: 248–254.
17. Scale Up to Process Chromatography (1983). Pharmacia Fine Chemicals, Uppsala, Sweden.
18. United States Pharmacopeia. (1985). 21st revision. United States Pharmacopeial Convention, Inc., p. 1187.
19. Juarez-Salinas, H., Engelhorn, S. C., Bigbee, W. L., Lowry, M. A., and Stanker, L. H. (1984). Ultrapurification of monoclonal antibodies by high-performance hydroxylapatite chromatography. *BioTechniques 2*: 164–168.
20. Stanker, L. H., Vanderlaan, M., and Juarez-Salinas, H. (1985). One-step purification of mouse monoclonal antibodies from ascites fluid by hydroxyapatite chromatography. *J. Immunol. Methods 76*: 157–169.
21. Lindmo, T., Boven, E., Cuttitta, F., Fedarko, J., and Bunn, P. A. (1984). Determination of the immunoreactive fraction of radiolabeled monoclonal antibodies by linear extrapolation to binding at infinite antigen excess. *J. Immunol. Methods 72*: 77–89.
22. Chaffotte, A. F., Djavadi-Ohaniance, L., and Goldberg, M. E. (1985). Does a monospecific hybridoma always secrete homogeneous immunoglobulins? *Biochimie 67*: 75–82.
23. Neville, D. M. Jr. and Glossmann, H. (1974). Molecular weight determination of membrane protein and glycoprotein subunits by discontinuous gel electrophoreses in dodecyl sulfate. In *Methods in Enzymology*, Vol. 32. Edited by S. Fleischer and L. Packer. New York, Academic Press, pp. 92–102.
24. Weber, K., Pringle, J. R., and Osborn, M. (1972). Measurement of molecular weights by electrophoresis on SDS-acrylamide gel. In *Methods in Enzymology*, Vol. 26. Edited by C. H. W. Hirs and S. N. Timasheff. New York, Academic Press, pp. 3–27.

25. Staines, N. A. (1983). Monoclonal antibodies. In *Biochemical Research Techniques.* Edited by J. M. Wrigglesworth. New York, John Wiley, pp. 177–209.

26. Duff, R. G. (1985). Microencapsulation technology: A novel method for monoclonal antibody production. *Trends Biotechnol. 3*: 167–170.

27. Leis, J. and Hurwitz, J. (1974). RNA-dependent DNA polymerase from avian myeloblastosis virus. In *Methods in Enzymology*, Vol. 29. Edited by L. Grossman and K. Moldave. New York, Academic Press, pp. 143–164.

28. Downs, T. R. and Wilfinger, W. W. (1983). Fluorometric quantification of DNA in cells and tissue. *Anal. Biochem. 131*: 538–547.

29. Zamora, P. O., Newell, K. D., Pant, K. D., Reed, K., and Rhodes, B. A. (1985). Production aspects of monoclonal antibodies for use in cancer radioimmunoimaging and therapy. *Am. Biotechnol. Lab. 3*: 50–57.

30. Chou, S. and Merigan, T. C. (1983). Rapid detection and quantitation of human cytomegalovirus in urine through DNA hybridization. *N. Engl. J. Med. 308*: 921–925.

31. Cuatrecasas, P., Wilchek, M., and Anfinsen, C. B. (1968). Selective enzyme purification by affinity chromatography. *Proc. Natl. Acad. Sci. U.S.A. 61*: 636–643.

32. Wilchek, M. and Miron, T. (1974). Polymers coupled to agarose as stable and high capacity spacers. In *Methods of Enzymology*, Vol. 34. Edited by W. B. Jakoby and M. Wilchek. New York, Academic Press, pp. 72–76.

33. Wilchek, M., Oka, T., and Topper, Y. J. (1975). Structure of a soluble superactive insulin is revealed by the nature of the complex between cyanogen bromide activated Sepharose and amines. *Proc. Natl. Acad. Sci. U.S.A. 72*: 1055–1058.

34. Dertzbaugh, M. T., Flickinger, M. C., and Lebherz, W. B. III. (1985). An enzyme immunoassay for the detection of staphylococcal protein A in affinity-purified products. *J. Immunol. Methods 83*: 169–177.

35. Goudswaard, J., Van Per Donk, J. A., Noordzij, A., Van Dam, R. H., and Vaerman, J. P. (1978). Protein A reactivity of various mammalian immunoglobulins. *Scand. J. Immunol. 8*: 21–28.

36. Dillman, R. O. and Royston, I. (1984). Applications of monoclonal antibodies in cancer therapy. *Br. Med. Bull. 40*: 240–246.

37. Underwood, P. A., Kelly, J. F., Harman, D. F., and MacMillan, H. M. (1983). Use of protein A to remove immunoglobulin from serum in hybridoma culture media. *J. Immunol. Methods 60*: 33–45.

38. Piotrowicz, B. I., Watt, I., Edlin, S., and McCartney, A. C. (1985). A micromethod for endotoxin assay in human plasma using limulus amoebocyte lysate and a chromogenic substrate. *Eur. J. Clin. Microbiol. 4*: 52–54.

39. Sofer, G. (1984). Chromatographic removal of pyrogens. *Biotechnology 2*: 1035–1038.

40. Morrison, D. C. and Ulevitch, R. J. (1978). The effects of bacterial endotoxins on host mediation systems. *Am. J. Pathol. 93*: 527–627.

41. Hou, K., Gerba, C. P., Goyal, S. M., and Zerda, K. S. (1980). Capture of latex beads, bacteria, endotoxin, and viruses by charge-modified filters. *Appl. Environ. Microbiol. 40*: 892–896.
42. Gerba, C. P., Hou, K. C., Babineau, R. A., and Fiore, J. V. (1980). Pyrogen control by depth filtration. *Pharm. Technol. 4*: 83–89.
43. Issekutz, A. C. (1983). Removal of gram-negative endotoxin from solutions by affinity chromatography. *J. Immunol. Methods 61*: 275–281.
44. Chibata, I., Tosa, T., Sato, T., Watanabe, T., and Minobe, S. (1983). Method for reducing the pyrogen content of or removing pyrogens from substances contaminated therewith. U.S. Patent 4,381,239.
45. Tutunjian, R. S. (1982). Pyrogen removal by ultrafiltration. *Prog. Clin. Biol. Res. 93*: 319–327.
46. Sweadner, K. J., Forte, M., and Nelsen, L. L. (1977). Filtration removal of endotoxin (pyrogens) in solution in different states of aggregation. *Appl. Environ. Microbiol. 34*: 382–385.
47. Grabner, R. W. (1975). Process for removing pyrogenic material from aqueous solutions. U.S. Patent 3,897,309.
48. Reichelderfer, P. S., Manischewitz, J. F., Wells, M. A., Hochstein, H. D., and Ennis, F. A. (1975). Reduction of endotoxin levels in influenza virus vaccines by barium sulfate adsorption-elution. *Appl. Microbiol. 30*: 333–334.
49. Nolan, J. P., McDevitt, J. J., and Goldmann, G. S. (1975). Endotoxin binding by charged and uncharged resins. *Proc. Soc. Exp. Biol. Med. 149*: 766–770.
50. Shadduck, R. K., Waheed, A., Porcellini, A., Rizzoli, V., and Levin, J. (1980). A method for the removal of endotoxin from purified colony-stimulating factor. *Proc. Soc. Exp. Biol. Med. 164*: 40–50.
51. Murray, G. J., Quirk, J. M., and Barranger, J. A. (1985). Removal of pyrogens from human β-hexosaminidase A by gel permeation HPLC. Fourth international symposium on HPLC of proteins, peptides, and polynucleotides. Abstract #219.
52. Kluger, M. J., Singer, R., and Eiger, S. M. (1985). Polymyxin B use does not ensure endotoxin-free solution. *J. Immunol. Methods 83*: 201–207.

12

Single-Step Purification of Monoclonal Antibodies by Anion Exchange High-Performance Liquid Chromatography

M. PATRICIA STRICKLER and M. JUDITH GEMSKI
Waters Chromatography Division, Millipore Corporation, Fairfax, Virginia

I. INTRODUCTION

The purification of monoclonal antibodies (MAb) from ascites and tissue culture supernatants is a crucial step in production. Two major factors must be considered. The first is that the separation technique yield MAb of consistent composition. The purity of MAb as well as the level of contaminants should always be within an acceptable range. To accomplish this, the composition of the crude sample (ascites or tissue culture) should be known prior to fractionation. The fractions arising from the separation of the crude sample should be monitored for composition prior to pooling.

The second major factor is the overall cost of the separation. A number of factors affect the cost of purification. The more obvious factors are the equipment, chromatographic media, reagents, and labor. There are, however, significant yet less obvious costs associated with a purification procedure. For example, a separation technique using a particular packing, column, and chromatographic unit may yield 1 g MAb/day, while another separation technique may yield 2-5 g MAb/day. Using the first technique would require two to five chromatographic units and columns to match the production of the latter separation. Effort spent in optimizing conditions may provide substantial savings in production costs.

There are, of course, many different ways to quantitate and monitor MAb levels, to develop and optimize production scale separations, and to control

217

the quality of product. Many of these techniques do not conveniently lend themselves to automation, quantitation, day-to-day reproducibility, high sensitivity, and production procedures. Also, many conventional separation techniques are slow and difficult to optimize. One technique that is quantitative, easily automated, reproducible, sensitive, and fast is high performance liquid chromatography (HPLC). In this chapter the use of ion exchange HPLC in the following areas will be discussed.

1. Qualitative and quantitative analysis of MAb and contaminating proteins in ascites and tissue culture supernatants
2. Development and optimization of chromatographic conditions for production scale separations (chromatographic process used to prepare MAb for market)
3. Qualitative and quantitative analysis of column fractions
4. Characterization of MAb
5. Determination of the maximum loading of sample on a column

The use of gel filtration HPLC coupled with high sensitivity detection will also be discussed for the qualitative and quantitative analysis of fractions generated by methods development and optimization separations, as well as production scale separations.

The production scale chromatographic unit need not be an HPLC. With some ion exchange chromatographic media an HPLC can be used for rapid, automated methods development while a peristaltic pump can be used in production scale separations. In either case a logical scale-up must be followed to maximize production and minimize costs.

II. PHYSICAL PROPERTIES OF ANION EXCHANGE MEDIA

A. Protein Pak DEAE-5PW

Two different anion exchange packings will be discussed for the purification of MAb. One exchanger is a 10 or 13 μm polymeric based weak anion exchanger with a 1000 Å pore. A diethylaminoethyl (DEAE) functionality is bonded to a polyether polymer. This packing, Protein Pak DEAE-5PW, is available only in prepacked analytical columns of 7.5 mm × 7.5 cm and 21 mm × 15 cm preparative columns. This packing is stable in the pH range 2-12 and can be made pyrogen free by washing with sodium hydroxide solutions. These columns, packed with microparticulate material, are designed to be run on HPLC equipment even though the back pressure generated by these columns is exceedingly low (less than 200 psi). This highly resolving column is ideally suited for the direct monitoring of MAb concentrations in ascites and tissue culture supernatants as well as the levels of contaminating proteins, especially other species of IgG.

B. ACCELL QMA

The other exchanger is a 40 μm encapsulated, silica-based, strong anion exchanger with a 500 Å pore. The silica is encapsulated with a hydrophilic bonded layer and a highly stable cross-linked functional layer containing the quaternary methylamine, QMA. The ACCELL QMA is stable in the pH range 2-9. The bulk packing can be sterilized by autoclaving the bulk packing as well as by washing with 0.1 N sodium hydroxide or hydrochloric acid to remove pyrogens after the column is packed. The 40 μm particle permits the user to pack any size column from analytical to production scale. The large particle size also allows the packing to be used with simple glass columns equipped with peristaltic pumps, as well as HPLC. The methods developed at the microgram level can then be applied to the same medium packed into a large preparative column.

III. SAMPLE PREPARATION

The preparation of the ascites and tissue culture fluid prior to a purification method is very important. Ideally, it should be simple and conservative of the MAb. The conventional preparation of an ascitic fluid for ion exchange chromatography has been either dialysis against the initial buffer or precipitation with ammonium sulfate to remove albumin, followed by dialysis. A simpler procedure is a 1/10 dilution of the ascites in the initial chromatographic buffer followed by filtration through a prewetted 0.45 μm membrane. Dilution lowers the salt concentration sufficiently to allow large volumes of filtrate to be applied directly to the column. Prewetting the filtration membrane with distilled water increases the volume that can be filtered. Tissue culture supernatant is diluted to one-third and filtered similarly. If the MAb concentration is very low, the supernatant may be concentrated by ultrafiltration prior to separation.

IV. MATERIALS AND METHODS

A. Ion Exchange Chromatography

Equipment for the ion exchange separations consisted of a pair of Waters model 510 solvent delivery systems, one of which was equipped with a three-way solvent inlet manifold for preparative loadings, a model U6K injector for analytical injections, and a model 481 variable wavelength ultraviolet detector. Gradients were generated either using a model 680 controller or a model 840 controller and computer. The chromatograms were recorded either on a strip chart recorder or with the model 840 controller and computer (Waters Chromatography Division, Millipore Corp., Milford, MA). The chromatographic packings used were either the Protein Pak DEAE-5PW prepacked in 7.5 mm X 7.5 cm and 21.5 mm X 15 cm columns (Waters), or the ACCELL QMA (Waters) slurry packed in a 7.5 mm X 7.5 cm stainless steel column or in a 25 mm X 25 cm glass column.

B. Gel Filtration Chromatography

The gel filtration HPLC system consisted of a Waters model 510 solvent delivery system, a model 441 ultraviolet detector set at 214 nm, a model 710B autosampler, and a model 840 controller and computer. Chromatography was carried out on either a pair of Protein Pak 300SW 7.8 mm X 30 cm columns or one Protein Pak 300SW and a Protein Pak 125 (7.8 mm X 30 cm) in series (Waters). One 300 SW column was also used for a more rapid analysis.

V. OPTIMIZATION OF CHROMATOGRAPHIC CONDITIONS

A. Standards

Ion exchange HPLC, because of its speed, is a convenient technique for developing and optimizing methods. A number of conditions can be evaluated rapidly using microgram amounts of commercially available immunoglobulin G, A, M and the major contaminating proteins transferrin and albumin. The MAb of interest may also be used, if available. One advantage of using standards is that fractions do not have to be collected and analyzed by some other technique to evaluate the separation. Variations in ionic strength and pH affect the elution of a protein from an ion exchange column. The optimal gradient conditions for the resolution of MAb were determined by running a series of standard proteins on the Protein Pak DEAE-5PW column (1). At a fixed pH, simple ionic strength gradients of NaCl could only resolve albumin from the standard mouse IgG. Ionic-strength gradients could not resolve IgG from transferrin. However, at pH 8.0 it was possible to separate IgA from IgG by an ionic-strength step gradient. Also, IgM could be resolved from albumin using step gradients. A series of pH gradients from 8.5 to 7.0, in 20 mm Tris buffer at a fixed ionic strength of 0.1 M NaCl, gave slight resolution of transferrin from IgG. IgA, albumin, and IgM were retained on the column under these conditions. At a fixed ionic strength of

0.15 M NaCl, IgG, IgA, and transferrin coeluted. Albumin and IgM, however, were still retained. When both pH and a shallow salt gradient were run simultaneously, good resolution of most of the proteins was obtained (Fig. 1). The standards IgG and IgA were not resolved using these conditions (IgA coelutes with IgG; not shown). However, an IgA MAb may be separable from polyclonal mouse IgG in the ascites and an IgG MAb from IgA present in the ascites. Likewise, using these optimized conditions it is possible in many cases to separate polyclonal mouse IgG present in the ascites from the IgG MAb. Phosphate buffers were not able to resolve the standard proteins as well as Tris buffers. Any optimization scheme should include at least two different buffer salts because the nature of the buffer may affect the selectivity of the separation.

B. Ascites

1. Immunoglobulin G Monoclonal Antibodies

Chromatographic conditions can also be optimized using the actual ascites or tissue culture fluid. Using the actual sample for optimization of conditions requires the collection of fractions and analysis by some other technique, such as gel filtration HPLC. Conditions were optimized in this fashion for the purification of monoclonal antibodies on a 7.5 mm × 7.5 cm column packed with ACCELL QMA (2). The resolution and recovery of MAb using the Tris pH and salt gradient were not as good as those achieved on the DEAE-5PW column. Variations in the pH of Tris buffer did not improve the separation.

Sodium phosphate buffers and linear NaCl gradients showed good resolution and recovery of an IgG_1 MAb from ascites (see Fig. 5B). Phosphate buffers in the pH range of 7.0 to 7.8 were tried on ACCELL QMA. Only pH 7.8 buffer failed to separate the MAb from transferrin and albumin. A pH of 7.0 was selected because it was possible to resolve polyclonal mouse IgG from the MAb.

The IgG MAbs generally separated well with the optimized conditions on both packings. With both packings, the resolution of transferrin from the IgG MAb was more difficult than resolution from albumin.

2. IgM MAbs

The purification of IgM monoclonals is more difficult because a generalized methodology has not yet been found. In contrast to the IgG MAbs, the resolution of albumin from IgM MAbs is more difficult. In some cases, the optimized conditions discussed previously work well and the IgM MAb will elute after albumin on the DEAE-5PW column. However, many IgM MAbs are not soluble in an initial buffer of 20 mm Tris. Conditions must be

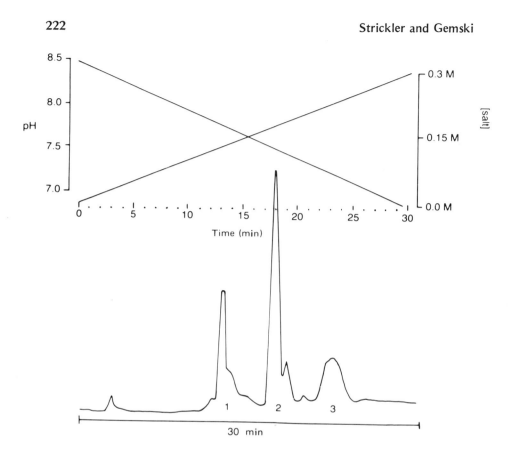

Figure 1 Optimal separation of standard proteins on the Protein Pak DEAE-5PW column. Chromatography was carried out on a 7.5 mm × 7.5 cm Protein Pak DEAE-5PW column using a 30 min linear gradient of 20 mM Tris, pH 8.5, to 20 mM Tris, pH 7.0, with 0.3 M NaCl at a flow rate of 1 ml/min. Standard proteins in a mixture of 25 μg human transferrin (peak 1), 50 μg mouse IgG (peak 2), and 25 μg bovine serum albumin (peak 3) were injected. Eluting peaks were monitored at 280 nm, 0.5 absorbance units full scale (AUFS).

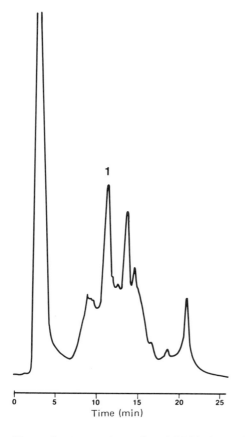

Figure 2 Separation of an IgM MAb on the Protein Pak DEAE-5PW column. Chromatography was carried out on a 7.5 mm × 7.5 cm Protein Pak DEAE-5PW column using a 30 min linear gradient of 20 mM Tris, pH 8.5, with 0.1 M NaCl to 20 mM Tris, pH 7.0, with 0.3 M NaCl at a flow rate of 1 ml/min. A 150 μl aliquot of partially purified IgM MAb (peak 1) from ascites was injected. Detection was at 280 nm, 0.1 AUFS.

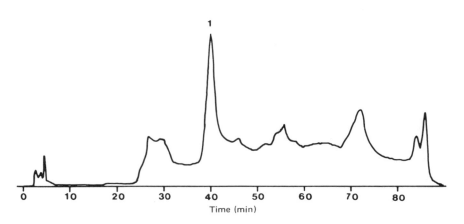

Figure 3   Separation of an IgM MAb on ACCELL QMA. Chromatography
was carried on a 7.5 mm X 7.5 cm column packed with ACCELL QMA
media using the following step ionic strength gradient containing 20 mM
sodium phosphate buffer, pH 7.0, at a flow rate of 0.5 ml/min: 0–15 min:
20 mM sodium phosphate, pH 7.0; 15–30 min: 20 mM sodium phosphate,
pH 7.0 + 0.1 M NaCl; 30–45 min: 20 mM sodium phosphate, pH 7.0 +
0.2 M NaCl; 45–60 min: 20 mM sodium phosphate, pH 7.0 + 0.3 M NaCl;
60–75 min: 20 mM sodium phosphate, pH 7.0 + 0.4 M NaCl.   A 200 μl
aliquot of partially purified IgM MAb (peak 1) was injected.   Detection was
at 280 nm, 0.05 AUFS.

modified to maintain the IgM in solution.   In fact, in some instances the
dilution of ascites containing the IgM MAb precipitates homogeneous IgM.
An example of a MAb run with a higher salt initial buffer is shown in Figure
2.   Under these modified conditions the recovered IgM MAb was contaminated with albumin.   A step gradient on the ACCELL QMA packing using
the pH 7.0 phosphate buffer gave superior resolution, as shown in Figure 3.
This example illustrates nicely that methods development and optimization
of chromatographic conditions prior to scale-up are important as well as
economical.   Scale-up on the DEAE-5PW column would be at least 20 times
more expensive for just the column packing alone.   The ACCELL QMA can
be run with a simple step gradient, which is easier than a continuous gradient
to generate reproducibly using a peristaltic pump.   Also, the use of this rigid
ion exchange medium rather than a soft gel ion exchanger will allow for a
faster separation: a few hours versus 12 hr.

C. Tissue Culture Supernatants

The same conditions used on the ascites can be applied to tissue culture, as well as serum-free media. Methods development on tissue culture supernatants is somewhat complicated by the presence of phenol red. This problem will be discussed in detail below.

VI. USE OF GEL FILTRATION HPLC FOR RAPID CONFIRMATION OF MAb PURITY

The optimization of chromatographic conditions is faster and more convenient if there is a rapid method of determining the identity and homogeneity of the ion exchange column fractions. Ideally, the method should be sensitive so that nanogram to microgram amounts of protein can be analyzed. It should also be quantitative and easy to automate since methods development and optimization experiments can generate many fractions. The monitoring of composition and confirmation of purity of a MAb from an ion exchange packing or any other chromatographic media can be rapidly accomplished using gel filtration HPLC. A Protein Pak 300SW column with 0.1 M sodium phosphate, pH 6.8, at a flow rate of 1 ml/min, can analyze a sample in 10 min. The column can be monitored at 280 nm or preferably at 214 nm. Detection at 214 nm is extremely sensitive and will detect impurities that could otherwise be seen only on a silver-stained polyacrylamide gel. Retention times of albumin, transferrin, and immunoglobulin G and M are summarized in Table 1. As little as 10 ng albumin and transferrin and 20 ng IgG can be detected by this technique. Fractions arising from the optimization experiment can be screened on an automated HPLC for MAb homogeneity. Up to six different chromatographic conditions can be tried in an 8-hr day and the resulting fractions run unattended overnight. If the automated HPLC is interfaced with an integrator or computer, quantitative data can also be obtained. Figure 4 illustrates the profile obtained from a series of fractions from the separation of an IgG$_1$ MAb from ascites. The first panel shows trace levels of MAb (retention time = 14.0 min) and transferrin (retention time = 15.0 min). The next two panels show high concentrations of MAb with no detectable transferrin or albumin. The bottom panel shows trace levels of MAb and high concentrations of albumin (retention time = 15.5 min). Since greater than 80% of the detectable MAb is free of contaminants, these separation conditions would certainly be adequate for scale-up. This information would determine which fractions should be pooled. A silver-stained polyacrylamide gel of the two homogeneous MAb fractions, #20 and #21, shows that greater than 93% of the stained material was MAb.

Table 1 Gel Filtration HPLC of Protein Standards

Protein standards	Retention time, 1-300SW (min)	Retention time, 1-300SW and 1-125 (min)	Minimum detectable level, 214 nm (ng)
Human transferrin	8.15	16.3	20
Bovine serum albumin	8.03	16.2	10
Mouse IgG	7.38	14.8	20
Mouse IgM (pentamer)	5.0	11.0	ND
Mouse IgM (monomer)	7.0	13.2	ND

The Protein Pak 300SW and 125 columns (Waters Chromatography Division, Millipore Corp., Milford, MA) are each 7.8 mm × 30 cm.

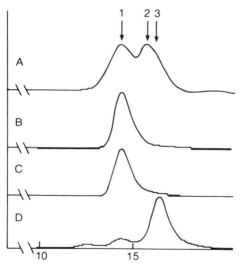

Time (min)

Figure 4 Gel filtration analyses of column fractions from the separation of 1 ml ascites on the Protein Pak DEAE-5PW column. Chromatography was carried out on two Protein Pak 300SW columns in series with a 0.1 M sodium phosphate buffer, pH 6.8, at a flow rate of 1 ml/min. The samples were monitored at 214 nm, 0.05 AUFS (panel A) and 1.0 AUFS (panels B, C, D). The elution positions of protein standards are shown by the numbered arrows above panel A for IgG (peak 1), transferrin (peak 2), and albumin (peak 3). Fractions correspond to the ion exchange separation shown in Figure 8. Panel A: column fraction #19; panel B: column fraction #20; panel C: column fraction #21; panel D: column fraction #23.

The IgM MAbs usually show two peaks by this technique. The higher-molecular-weight peak elutes at the exclusion volume of the column and corresponds to the pentamer. A second peak elutes before IgG and corresponds to the "monomer." It is interesting that the relative sizes of these two peaks vary greatly from one IgM MAb to another.

Since gel filtration HPLC can rapidly monitor the composition of a fraction, it can be used to analyze and quantify MAb in the fractions from the production scale separations prior to pooling fractions. All of this can occur unattended.

VII. MAb PURIFICATION FROM ASCITES FLUID

With use of the optimized chromatographic system on the Protein Pak DEAE-5PW, samples of ascites containing a variety of MAbs can be analyzed rapidly for protein composition and the amount of MAb present. For example, a MAb may have different heavy and light chain combinations, not all of which are equally active. Examination on the DEAE-5PW column will show heterogeneity of the MAb and, in some instances, resolve the different forms. The individual species can be isolated and the relative activity and specificity of each species determined (3). This technique can also allow various MAbs raised to the same antigen to be screened for ease of purification. The concentration of MAb being produced in the ascites can also be monitored and quantified. The levels of contaminating proteins, transferrin and albumin, specifically, relative to the concentration of MAb can also be monitored. For example, transferrin levels in the mouse are variable. Therefore, monitoring the transferrin level as well as the MAb level would show if the production scale separation conditions needed modification to eliminate elevated transferrin levels. A comparison of the retention times on both the DEAE-5PW and the ACCELL QMA of the major components present in representative ascites is summarized in Table 2. There is no standard retention time for all MAbs, even MAbs of the same subtype. An example of the separation of the same ascites on both packings is shown in Figure 5.

The DEAE-5PW column can also be used to assess the homogeneity of fractions from methods development and optimization of conditions from other packing materials. For example, as mentioned previously in the section on Optimization, polyclonal mouse IgG can usually be separated from MAb on the DEAE-5PW column. Therefore, if the removal of host IgG is desired, this column could be used to assay MAb fractions for mouse IgG contamination. Gel filtration HPLC will not show the presence of mouse IgG, since IgG will coelute with IgG MAb.

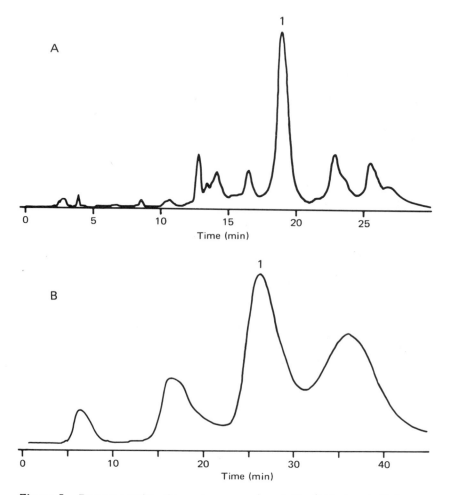

Figure 5 Representative chromatograms of an IgG_1 MAb (peak 1) from ascites on Protein Pak DEAE-5PW and ACCELL QMA. Panel A: The separation of 200 μl of a 1:20 dilution of ascites on a Protein Pak DEAE-5PW 7.5 mm X 7.5 cm column using the optimal conditions described in Figure 1. Detection was at 280 nm, 0.15 AUFS. Panel B: The separation of 500 μl of a 1:20 dilution of ascites on a 7.5 mm X 7.5 cm column packed with ACCELL QMA using a 45 min linear gradient from 20 mM sodium phosphate buffer, pH 7.0 to 20 mM sodium phosphate buffer, pH 7.0, with 0.4 M NaCl at a flow rate of 0.5 ml/min. Eluting peaks were monitored at 280 nm, 0.13 AUFS.

Table 2   Retention Times of Representative IgG MAbs, Transferrin, and
Albumin from Ascites

IgG subtype	Retention time MAbs DEAE-5PW[a] (min)	Retention time MAbs ACCELL QMA[b] (min)
IgG$_1$	21.0	24.0
IgG$_1$	18.8	27.1
IgG$_{2b}$	18.4	29.3
IgG$_{2a}$	16.1	21.0
IgG$_1$	17.1	22.2
IgG$_1$	16.2	21.0
IgG$_3$	14.1	18.5
Transferrin	13.0	17.5
Albumin	23.0	36.5

[a]The Protein Pak DEAE-5PW column, 7.5 mm × 7.5 cm (Waters). A 30 min linear
gradient of 20 mm Tris, pH 8.5, to 20 mm Tris, pH 7.0, with 0.3 M NaCl at 1 ml/min
was run.
[b]A 7.5 mm × 7.5 cm column packed with ACCELL QMA (Waters). A 45 min linear
gradient of 20 mm sodium phosphate, pH 7.0, to 20 mm sodium phosphate, pH 7.0,
with 0.4 M NaCl at 0.5 ml/min was run.

VIII. MAb PURIFICATION FROM TISSUE CULTURE SUPERNATANTS

A. Effect of Phenol Red on MAb Separations

Hybridoma cells grown in tissue culture fluids present additional problems for
recovery by ion exchange chromatography due to the presence of phenol red
indicator in the culture medium. Phenol red (phenolsulfonphthalein) binds
to the anion exchanger DEAE-5PW at salt concentrations less than 1.0 M
NaCl. The pH indicator modifies the column chemistry and limits the
capacity of the column for purifying MAb from tissue culture supernatants.
The elution position of a MAb is the same when the hybridoma is grown in
ascites or tissue culture, as shown in Figure 6. The additional complication
of phenol red in the media can be seen in Figure 6, panel B, in the broadening
of the MAb and albumin peaks. Phenol red binds to the DEAE-5PW column
under these chromatographic conditions. It can be washed from the column
with 1.0 M NaCl. The ACCELL QMA packing does not seem to bind the

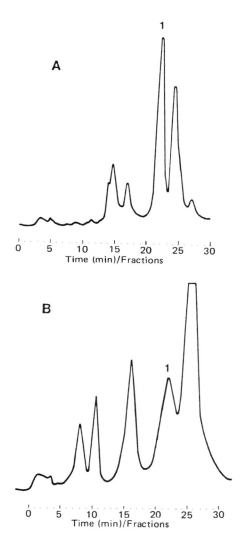

Figure 6 Separation of an IgG$_1$ MAb from ascites and tissue culture fluids. Panel A: A 50 μl aliquot of an IgG$_1$ MAb (peak 1) in a 1:20 dilution of ascites on the Protein Pak DEAE-5PW 7.5 mm $\times$ 7.5 cm column using the optimal conditions described previously in Figure 1. The detector was set at 280 nm, 0.5 AUFS. Panel B: A 1 ml aliquot of the same MAb (1) shown in panel A in a 1:3 dilution of tissue culture supernatant using the conditions described above.

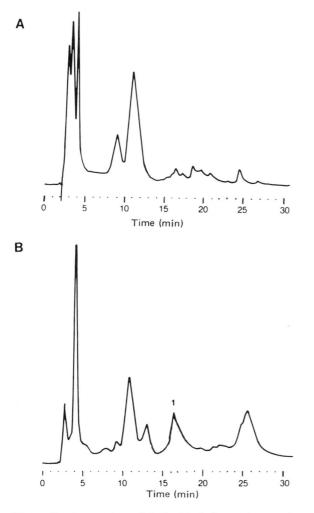

Figure 7   Separation of IgG_1 MAb from tissue culture supernatant grown in serum-free media.   Panel A: Injection of 250 μl Iscove's serum-free media diluted 1:3 with water on the Protein Pak DEAE-5PW 7.5 mm $\times$ 7.5 cm column using the optimal conditions described in Figure 1.   Panel B: Injection of 250 μl of the above medium containing an IgG_1 MAb (peak 1). The detector was set at 280 nm, 0.05 AUFS in both panels.

phenol red as does the DEAE-5PW as evidenced by the absence of band broadening (results not shown).

Phenol red also binds very strongly to protein. The MAb as well as immunoglobulin standards in the presence of phenol red show a significant shift in retention time (0.5 min) on the gel filtration HPLC columns. After removal of phenol red as judged by the absence of color, this same shift in retention time is still noted. The small amounts of phenol red that remain bound to the protein may produce problems in the end use of a MAb. If phenol red were not present in the media, the purification of MAb from tissue culture supernatants would be a very simple separation and large volumes of supernatant could be applied directly to the column. Since there are many other ways to monitor pH, it is the authors' recommendation to purchase media without phenol red, or at least to examine the phenol red issue prior to establishing a production procedure.

B. Serum-Free Medium

Monoclonal antibodies grown in serum-free media are purified using the same technique. Figure 7 shows an example of a separation of serum-free media (panel A) and an IgG_1 MAb grown in the serum-free media (panel B). Panel A emphasizes the point that any optimization of conditions from tissue culture must include chromatography of the medium since this will contribute several peaks.

The MAb concentration in tissue culture supernatant can also be monitored and quantified on the Protein Pak DEAE-5PW column. This can be very useful in choosing the conditions for maximum production of MAb from the tissue culture. The quality of the fetal calf serum used in the growth medium can also easily be monitored using the same column and chromatographic conditions. The amount of calf IgG varies significantly. A serum with very low levels of IgG makes purification easier.

IX. SCALE-UP CONSIDERATIONS

A. Determination of the Maximum Sample Amount in the Production Scale Separation

Once the chromatographic conditions have been optimized at the analytical level with microgram quantities of sample, the maximum column loading of sample can be determined. A loading study carried out on the analytical column will not only maximize load while maintaining the desired purity levels but also reveal any problems that might be associated with loading a large sample. Common problems are shifts in retention times, peak skewing, and loss of recovery due to solubility limitations. Figure 8 is an example of a loading study performed on the analytical DEAE-5PW column with ascites at a protein concentration of 30 mg/ml. A slight loss in resolution between the MAb and albumin is seen with a loading of 0.5 ml ascites (panel C). Application of 1 ml ascites (panel D) shows no resolution between the MAb and albumin and a decrease in retention times. Analysis of the fractions from the separation of 1 ml ascites (panel D) by gel filtration HPLC shows fractions 20 and 21 to be free from any transferrin contamination as seen in fraction 19, and any albumin contamination as in fraction 23 (Fig. 4). This series of chromatograms exemplifies the need to analyze the fractions from a separation when resolution in the chromatogram is no longer discernable. Figure 8, panel D, shows no resolution between MAb and albumin; however by gel filtration, shown in Figure 4, fraction 21 shows a clear separation from albumin. The MAb in fractions 20 and 21 is recovered 93% pure (determined by silver-stained SDS gel electrophoresis). Fractions 20 and 21 represent greater than 80% of the MAb recovered from the separation. Further experiments indicated that the total protein load for an 80% recovery of pure MAb is 50 mg. If a lower recovery of homogeneous MAb in a single step were acceptable or if the purity requirements were less stringent than in this example, more ascites could be applied to the column.

The total recovery of MAb from this column can also be estimated by integrating the MAb peak area and plotting the total peak area recovered versus the volume of ascites injected. Figure 9 shows the mass recovery of MAb from this loading study. If the plot were not linear, it would indicate nonspecific binding of the protein or precipitation of the protein on the column. It is possible to exceed the solubility of the protein as it is concentrated at the head of the column.

A similar loading study was performed on the ACCELL QMA packed in a 7.5 mm × 7.5 cm column. The maximum protein load for the same ascites, recovering 80% of the MAb homogeneous, was 10 mg. Particle size influences the amount of sample that can be loaded because it affects the efficiency of the packing. Since the ACCELL QMA has a 40 μm particle compared to the 10 μm DEAE-5PW, less ascites can be loaded onto the same size columns packed with 40 μm compared to 10 μm material.

B. Determination of Direct Scale-Up Parameters

Once the maximum loading of ascites on the analytical column has been determined, the amount of sample that can be injected onto the preparative column can be calculated using Eq. (1).

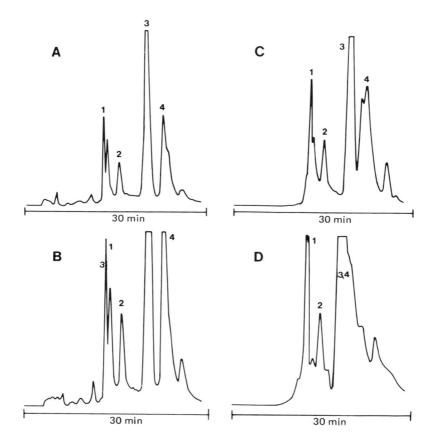

Figure 8 Maximum sample amount loading study on the analytical Protein Pak DEAE-5PW column. Chromatography was carried out on the 7.5 mm X 7.5 cm column using the optimal conditions described in Figure 1. All ascites were diluted 1:20 with the initial buffer and filtered. Injection volumes greater than 2 ml were applied to the column directly through the pump. Transferrin (peak 1), polyclonal mouse IgG (peak 2), IgG_1 MAb (peak 3), and albumin (peak 4) are shown. Panel A: Detection at 280 nm, 0.05 AUFS; injection volume 1.0 ml or 0.05 ml ascites. Panel B: Detection at 280 nm, 0.05 AUFS; injection volume 2.0 ml or 0.1 ml ascites. Panel C: Detection at 280 nm, 2.0 AUFS; injection volume 10 ml or 0.5 ml ascites. Panel D: Detection at 280 nm, 2.0 AUFS; injection volume 20 ml or 1 ml ascites.

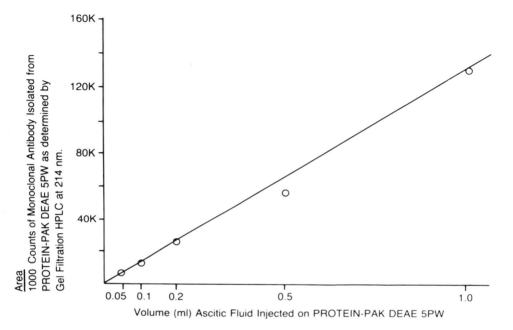

Figure 9 Mass recovery of MAb from Portein Pak DEAE-5PW. The mass of MAb recovered, quantified by peak areas from gel filtration HPLC, is plotted against the amount of ascites injected on the DEAE-5PW column. Linearity indicates a quantitative recovery of MAb with increasing sample loads.

$$\text{Preparative (prep.) sample amount} = \text{Analytic sample amount} \times \frac{(D_2)^2 \times L_2}{(D_1)^2 \times L_1}$$

$$(1)$$

where D_2 = diameter of prep. column, L_2 = length of prep. column, D_1 = diameter of analytic column, L_1 = length of analytic column.

Therefore, 16 ml ascites (30 mg/ml) or 480 mg is the preparative sample loading on the 21.5 mm × 15 cm DEAE-5PW column. Since the ACCELL QMA can be packed into any size column, the amount of sample to be fractionated would determine the column dimensions. If a 25 mm × 25 cm glass column packed with ACCELL QMA were used, 12 ml ascites or 360 mg protein could be applied to the column.

The flow rate of the preparative column is calculated using Eq. (2).

$$\text{Flow rate prep.} = \text{Flow rate anal.} \times \frac{(D_2)^2}{(D_1)^2} \qquad (2)$$

The calculated flow rates for the preparative DEAE-5PW and the ACCELL QMA would be 8 ml/min and 5.5 ml/min, respectively.

Another factor to be determined is the duration of the gradient. If the analytical and preparative columns were of equal lengths, the gradient time on the preparative column would be the same as on the analytical column. In this case the column lengths are different and the gradient duration must be calculated using Eq. (3).

$$\text{Gradient duration prep.} = \frac{(D_2)^2 \ L_2 \times \text{Gradient duration anal.} \times \text{Flow rate anal.}}{(D_1)^2 \ L_1 \times \text{Flow rate prep.}}$$

$$\qquad (3)$$

The duration of the gradient on the DEAE-5PW and ACCELL QMA columns would be 60 min and 150 min, respectively. The direct scale-up of the analytical conditions to the preparative column would employ the same buffers with the calculated gradient durations and flow rates.

C. Repetitive Injection Chromatography

Using direct scale-up, 480 mg protein could be injected every 90 min on the preparative DEAE-5PW: 60 min for the separation, 15 min for reequilibration, and 15 min for sample loading. Based on an 8-hr day, 2.4 g protein could be processed per day, yielding approximately 800 mg MAb (concentration of MAb = 10 mg/ml). This procedure could be automated to increase production. Using the ACCELL QMA 25 mm × 25 cm column, 360 mg protein could be loaded every 180 min for a total of 1.0 g protein processed per day, yielding 360 mg MAb. A cost comparison of the two packings shows the DEAE-5PW packing to be 20 times more expensive than the ACCELL QMA, approximately $2000.00 versus $100.00.

Production scale separations can be performed either by repetitive injections on a small preparative column, as discussed previously, or by injection of the whole sample on one large column. The choice of methodology would depend on the amount of MAb required over time. For example, if 2 g MAb were required every month, the repetitive injection procedure would certainly be adequate and economical. Two to 4 days a month could be spent in production. However, if 2 g MAb were required each day, a much larger column would be required.

X. REALITIES OF SCALE-UP

Resolution and recovery of MAb can be accurately predicted using a direct scale-up strategy. However, the direct scale-up may not be the most productive or the most economical. For example, less than optimal amounts of sample may be available for injection on an existing column. In this case, the gradient duration and flow rate may be adjusted to use less buffer, as shown in Figure 10, panels A and B. Aliquots of 0.5 and 5.0 ml ascites were applied to the column through the solvent inlet manifold of the pump and the gradient was initiated after loading. Panel A shows that in the separation of 0.5 ml ascites, the MAb (retention time = 39 min) is "baseline resolved" from albumin. The 5.0 ml aliquot of ascites (panel B) shows resolution between MAb and albumin similar to that of the 0.5 ml ascites separation in Figure 9, panel C. The comparable resolution between the 0.5 ml injection on the analytical column and the 5.0 ml injection on the preparative column indicates that with a 60 min gradient at 4 ml/min, rather than the calculated 8 ml/min, the maximum sample amount that could be injected on the preparative column is 10 times that for the analytical column rather than 16 times, as predicted by Eq. (1).

Gel filtration HPLC and SDS gel analyses of the fractions from Figure 10 indicated that the MAb is recovered with a high degree of homogeneity (1). On silver staining, trace amounts of protein bands were visualized, with MAb accounting for greater than 93% of the stained material. A calculation of mass recovery determined by gel filtration analysis indicated 90% of the expected yield based on the analytical loading study.

A 2 ml aliquot of this same ascites was applied to a preparative glass column (25 mm × 25 cm) packed with ACCELL QMA. The results are illustrated in Figure 11. Panel A shows the separation of 25 μl ascites on the analytical column (7.5 mm × 7.5 cm), while panel B shows 80 times that amount (2 ml) on the preparative column. The resolution of MAb and albumin is similar on the preparative and the analytical columns. The calculated scale factor for these column dimensions is close to 40X (Eq. 1), but by increasing the length of the gradient from 150 to 165 min and running at 2 ml/min the maximum sample amount is increased from 12 to 24 ml ascites. This shows that the loading on a preparative column can be increased over the calculated direct scale-up by extending the duration of the gradient. Modification of the chromatographic conditions from the direct scale-up

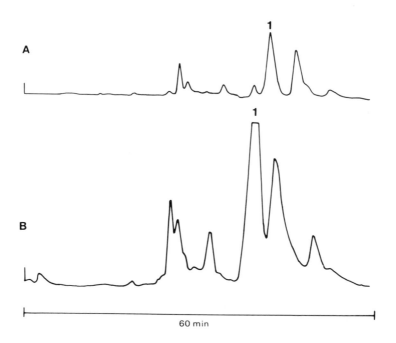

Figure 10   Preparative scale isolation of an IgG_1 MAb (peak 1) from ascites. Chromatography was carried out using a 21.5 mm $\times$ 15 cm Protein Pak DEAE-5PW column using a 60 min linear gradient from 20 mM Tris, pH 8.5, to 20 mM Tris, pH 7.0, with 0.3 M NaCl at a flow rate of 4 ml/min. Detection was at 280 nm, 2.0 AUFS. Panel A: 0.5 ml ascites diluted 1:20 with initial buffer. Panel B: 5.0 ml ascites diluted 1:20 with initial buffer.

values will increase the maximum loading of sample. In this case, a 15-min increase in gradient duration doubled the maximum sample loading.

SDS gel analysis and gel filtration HPLC confirmed the homogeneity of the MAb fractions. In addition, each fraction containing MAb was analyzed on the analytical DEAE-5PW column to verify if the MAb IgG_1 was free of host mouse IgG (Fig. 12). In this separation, host mouse IgG elutes at 16 min while MAb IgG_1 elutes at 22 min; transferrin and albumin elute at 13 and 25 min, respectively.

Recovery of biological activity was greater than 95% in 14 of 15 different ascites (1). In at least 5 other ascites, activity was recovered but not quantitated.

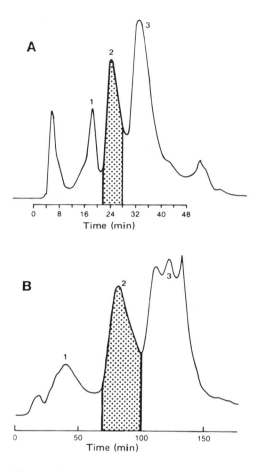

Figure 11   Preparative scale-up study of IgG$_1$ MAb on ACCELL QMA.
Transferrin (peak 1), IgG$_1$ MAb (peak 2), and albumin (peak 3) are shown.
Panel A: Separation of 25 μl ascites diluted 1:20 on ACCELL QMA packed
in a 7.5 mm X 7.5 cm column using a 45 min linear gradient of 20 mM
sodium phosphate, pH 7.0 to 20 mM sodium phosphate, pH 7.0, with 0.4 M
NaCl at a flow rate of 0.5 ml/min. Detection was at 280 nm, 0.2 AUFS.
Panel B: Separation of 2 ml ascites diluted 1:20 on ACCELL QMA packed in
a 25 mm X 25 cm column using a 165 min linear gradient of 20 mM sodium
phosphate, pH 7.0, to 20 mM sodium phosphate, pH 7.0, with 0.4 M NaCl
at a flow rate of 2 ml/min. Detection was at 280 nm, 1.0 AUFS.

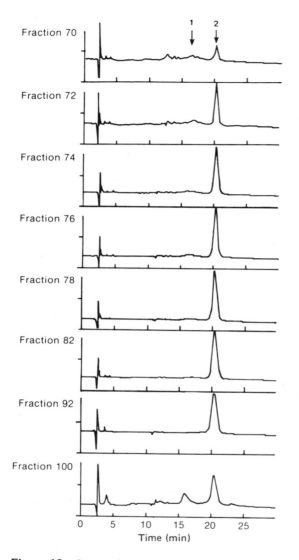

Figure 12   Ion exchange analyses of fractions from the preparative ACCELL QMA column. Chromatography was carried out on the Protein Pak DEAE-5PW 7.5 mm X 7.5 cm column using the optimal conditions described in Figure 1. One hundred μl of each of the fractions containing MAb from the preparative ACCELL QMA separation (Fig. 11) were injected. Detection was at 280 nm, 0.08 AUFS. Polyclonal mouse IgG elutes at position 1 and IgG_1 MAb at position 2.

XI. PREPARATIVE ISOLATION AND RECOVERY OF MAb FROM TISSUE CULTURE SUPERNATANTS

Preparative scale isolations from tissue culture supernatants are complicated by the presence of phenol red in the media. As previously discussed, phenol red binds to the DEAE-5PW packing and is not eluted with less than 1.0 M NaCl. The presence of phenol red on the column broadens the protein peaks. However, this in itself would not pose a serious problem other than the need to wash the column after each run. The low levels of MAb secreted in tissue culture require that large volumes of supernatant be applied to the column. A 14 ml aliquot of tissue culture supernatant was applied to the 21 mm × 15 cm DEAE-5PW column. The resulting chromatogram is shown in Figure 13, top panel. The MAb peak at 39 min has a shoulder at 37 min that did not occur in the analytical separation (Fig. 6, panel A). Gel filtration HPLC showed this peak, as well as a series of unresolved peaks at approximately 30 min, to be protein with the same retention time as the bovine IgG standard. Analyses of these fractions on the analytical DEAE-5PW column are shown in Figure 13, lower panels. Fraction 30 from the preparative separation elutes as a single peak on the analytical DEAE-5PW column at 16 min, corresponding to the retention time of the IgG standard, while fraction 37 from the preparative column is a mixture of the 16-min IgG peak and the 21-min MAb. Fraction 39 from the preparative column is homogeneous MAb, as seen on the analytical DEAE-5PW column. The shoulder at 37 min in the preparative separation is IgG from the calf serum present in the medium. Besides broadening the protein peaks, the phenol red also alters the chromatography, causing a portion of the calf serum IgG to elute at 37 min. This phenomenon reduces the capacity of the column.

In another case, the phenol red was removed from a concentrated tissue culture supernatant containing an IgG_{2a} MAb prior to scale-up by applying the supernatant (50 ml) directly to the preparative DEAE-5PW column. The protein was eluted in one fraction with 20 mM Tris, pH 8.5, 0.3 M NaCl. As expected, the phenol red bound to the packing. The eluted fraction (25 ml) containing all the protein was diluted to 150 ml and reapplied to the preparative DEAE-5PW column after the phenol red had been eluted with 1 M NaCl. The protein then fractionated as shown in Figure 14, panel A. These fractions analyzed on the analytical DEAE-5PW column showed the MAb to be free of calf serum IgG (panel B).

In this laboratory, large-scale separations of the proteins in tissue culture supernatants on the ACCELL QMA have not been attempted to date, although separations of MAb from tissue culture supernatant on analytical columns have not shown any interference from phenol red.

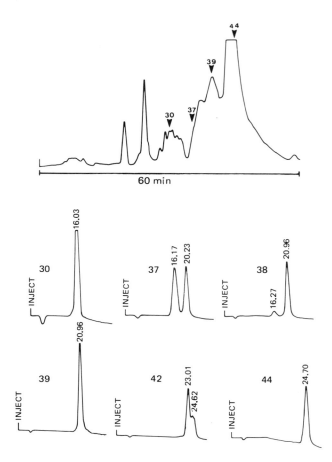

Figure 13 Preparative scale chromatography of MAb from tissue culture fluid in the presence of phenol red. Chromatography was carried out as described in Figure 10 using a preparative size column (21.5 mm × 15 cm) at 4 ml/min, monitored at 280 nm, 1.0 AUFS. Top panel: Injection of 14 ml tissue culture supernatant containing an IgG$_1$ MAb diluted to 42 ml with the initial conditions buffer. Fractions were collected every minute and numbered according to their elution time. Fractions 30, 37, 39, and 44 are indicated by arrows. Bottom panels: Rechromatography of fractions 30, 37, 38, 39, 42, and 44 on a 7.5 mm × 7.5 cm Protein Pak DEAE-5PW column as described in Figure 1. Detection was at 280 nm, 0.1 AUFS. The calf serum IgG elutes at 16.1 min, the IgG$_1$ MAb elutes at 20.1 min, and albumin elutes at 24.7 min.

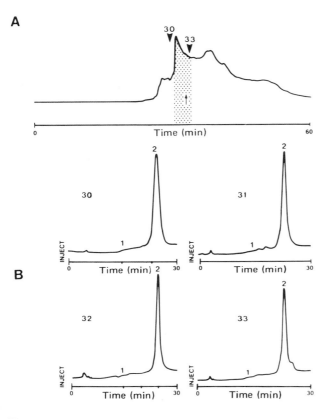

Figure 14 Preparative scale separation of an IgG_{2a} MAb from tissue culture supernatant after removal of phenol red. A 50 ml aliquot of tissue culture supernatant diluted 1:3 with 20 mM Tris, pH 8.5, was injected onto the 21.5 mm × 15 cm Protein Pak DEAE-5PW column in 20 mM Tris, pH 8.5, with 0.3 M NaCl. A 25 ml aliquot containing all the protein but with most of the phenol red removed was collected and diluted to 150 ml with 20 mM Tris, pH 8.5. Panel A: Chromatography of 150 ml of the diluted fraction from the above procedure. Separation conditions are described in Figure 10. The column was monitored at 254 nm, 0.6 AUFS, with a semipreparative flow cell. Fractions were collected every minute and numbered according to their elution time. Fractions 30–33 (shaded area) contain the MAb. Panel B: Rechromatography of fractions 30–33 from the above separation on the Protein Pak DEAE-5PW 7.5 mm × 7.5 cm column using the conditions described in Figure 1. The MAb (peak 2) is free of calf serum IgG (peak 1). Detection was at 280 nm, 0.1 AUFS.

XII. SUMMARY

HPLC is a valuable and powerful tool for both research and production of MAb. In conjunction with packing materials, such as Protein Pak DEAE-5PW, it can be used for rapid screening of ascites and microisolations of MAb. A series of MAbs can be characterized and evaluated before one is chosen for production. The levels of MAb produced in ascites or tissue culture can also be reliably quantified. The DEAE-5PW in conjunction with the gel filtration column can be used as an analytical technique for determining the homogeneity of MAb fractions from methods development and optimization experiments as well as from production scale purifications. Since HPLC is easily automated, many fractions can be analyzed reproducibly and the concentrations of MAb and contaminating proteins quantified reliably.

The ACCELL QMA media can be used for large-scale production separations using either a HPLC or an open-column equipped with a peristaltic pump. Because it is rigid, this packing can be operated at higher flow rates than soft gels such as Sepharose, Sephacel, or cellulose, to decrease the total separation time. Faster separation times allow the possibility of a greater number of repetitive injection purifications, thus increasing the overall yield of MAb from each chromatographic unit. HPLC can be used to determine the optimal chromatographic conditions and screen many packings and buffers for optimal MAb purification. Rapid determination of the optimal separation parameters is one of the greatest advantages HPLC offers. The choice of the most productive methodology will affect the entire manufacturing operation. Once chosen, it is difficult and costly to change.

ACKNOWLEDGMENTS

We wish to thank Dr. B. P. Doctor and Mary Kay Gentry, Walter Reed Army Institute of Research, Washington, D.C.; Dr. David Klapper, University of North Carolina School of Medicine, Chapel Hill, N.C.; Dr. John Maples, Naval Medical Research Center, Bethesda, MD; Dr. Charles Birdwell, Hybritech, San Diego, CA; Dr. Sally Seaver, Hygeia, Newton, MA; and Dr. Malcolm Pluskal and Dr. Joseph Gabriels, Millipore Corp., Bedford, MA, for supplying samples and technical assistance. We also wish to thank Betsy Baer, Waters, Fairfax, VA for editing the manuscript.

REFERENCES

1. Gemski, M. J., Doctor, B. P., Gentry, M. K., Pluskal, M. G., and Strickler, M. P. (1985). Single step purification of monoclonal antibody from

murine ascites and tissue culture fluids by anion exchange high performance liquid chromatography. *BioTechniques 3*: 387–384.

2. Strickler, M. P. and Gemski, M. J. (1986). Protein purification on a new preparative ion exchanger. *J. Liquid Chromatogr. 9*(8): 1655–1677.

3. Unpublished data.

13

ABx: A Novel Chromatographic Matrix for the Purification of Antibodies

DAVID R. NAU
J. T. Baker Chemical Company, Phillipsburg, New Jersey

I. INTRODUCTION

The purification of antibodies is one of the oldest challenges in protein bio-chemistry. Even today, despite a long history of use of antibodies as tools for analysis, identification, characterization, and purification, the development of rapid and economical purification schemes for antibodies remains a major problem for research and production personnel. Recently, these purification problems have become even more acute. The primary reason for this dilemma is that the development of monoclonal antibody technology (1), by providing an enormous impetus for progress in numerous fields of science and technology (2), has created new and more demanding purification problems. Large quantities of high-purity nonpyrogenic immunoglobulin are now required for in vivo diagnostics (imaging) and immunotherapeutics (3,4), for use in affinity chromatography for the purification of pharmaceuticals (5,6), and, to a lesser extent, for in vitro diagnostic kits (7,8).

Prior to the advent of monoclonal antibodies the universal source of immunoglobulins was serum/plasma. Since IgGs typically represent a major portion of the total protein complement of serum, rigorous purification was often not essential for the intended use. The major concern was usually the elimination of nonspecific interactions rather than absolute product purity. Furthermore, the in vivo use of antibody preparations was rarely, if ever, attempted.

247

However, present trends favor using hybridoma cell cultures to produce large amounts of antibody. This is despite the fact that the levels of antibody are 2-3 orders of magnitude lower in culture supernatants than in ascites fluid or serum. Furthermore, most cells are cultured in the presence of fetal calf serum or horse serum that contains high levels of many different types of proteins (9-11). Even in serum-free hybridoma tissue culture medium, where the protein complement is not extremely complex, the purification may nonetheless be difficult because the monoclonal antibody is often present as a minor component. In the case of ascites fluids, contaminating proteins may also consist of "host" polyclonal antibodies, while fetal bovine sera also contain low levels (40-400 µg/ml) of bovine serum immunoglobulins (9-14).

In addition, antibody purification is no longer limited to IgG, since numerous monoclonals of therapeutic interest are now IgMs and other immunoglobulin classes. Furthermore, as techniques for hybridoma manipulation and immunochemistry become increasingly sophisticated, new purification procedures are needed for cell lines secreting multiple immunoglobulins, bivalent hybrid antibodies, protein-antibody conjugates, antibody fragments, hybrid fragments, and chemically modified monoclonals (15). Therefore, antibody purification is not one problem but many.

As a result, purification methods are constantly being scrutinized and optimized to achieve more homogeneous antibody preparations. Unfortunately, most of the approaches to immunoglobulin purification currently in use are simply variations of the long-established purification procedures for serum polyclonal antibodies.

II. TRADITIONAL ANTIBODY PURIFICATION

Preparative-scale antibody purification has traditionally been carried out on biopolymer-based DEAE-type soft gels which are based upon polysaccharides and other polymers such as cellulose, dextrans, agarose, or polyacrylamides (16-18). Although anion exchange chromatography on soft gels requires simple equipment, can be scaled-up to a certain extent, and produces antibodies at a purity adequate for a number of end uses, traditional soft gels suffer from a number of serious disadvantages as general preparative-scale purification tools. Most importantly, soft gels provide extremely low resolution between antibodies and contaminating proteins such as albumins and transferrins. Chromatography must typically be combined with an initial ammonium sulfate salt fractionation step (16-18). Soft gels have inherently low capacities for binding proteins. Thus, large quantities of gel and extremely long chromatographic run times are required to achieve adequate separations. In addition, high flow rates, which are desirable in preparative chromatography for high throughput and rapid reequilibration and regeneration, are not possible on soft gels due to high back pressures, poor mechanical strength, and the possibility of column collapse. The life expectancy of soft gels is also rather short. It is often tempting to discard the matrix after each use, because of the cumbersome maintenance and regeneration procedures and the fact that polysaccharide based gels themselves support the growth of microorganisms. This biodegradability, as well as chemical instability and difficulty in sterilization, lead to the possibility of contamination of the final antibody preparation by endotoxin and degradation product. Finally, soft gels tend to bind immunoglobulin irreversibly, which decreases yield and the overall economics of the purification.

III. MODERN ANTIBODY PURIFICATION

A. High-Performance Anion Exchange Chromatography

Recent work in our laboratories and in those of others, indicates that chromatography on high-performance anion exchange matrices may provide a useful approach to monoclonal antibody purification (9-12,19-23) since these materials overcome many of the problems inherent in soft gels. Most importantly, these HPLC materials give much higher resolution than traditional matrices. Furthermore, the capacity of these matrices is typically much higher than those of soft gels; they can bind as much as 150 mg purified IgG/g packing (9-11). These factors, combined with the ability to use higher flow rates, allow for substantially higher throughput on much smaller columns. Finally, HPLC supports tend to be much more rugged than soft gels, allowing longer column lifetime and increased chemical stability.

Although substantial progress has recently been made in the area of monoclonal antibody purification, it has become increasingly apparent that the purification of monoclonal antibodies by high-performance anion exchange chromatographic matrices also has several limitations. The "background" profiles of contaminating nonimmunoglobulin proteins tend to vary considerably depending upon species, strain, and individual hybridoma. More importantly, individual monoclonals may elute at a wide range of retention times within the gradient (9-11,21,22,24), thereby reducing the possibility of achieving homogeneous antibody, and making method development and identification of the antibody peak difficult. The binding of dyes (i.e., phenol red) decreases resolution by broadening the antibody and albumin peaks and changes the elution characteristics of the immunoglobulin peaks because it changes the mechanism of the separation (9-12,24). These dyes also dramatically reduce the ability of the anion exchange matrices to bind protein to a mere fraction of their original capacity (9-12,24). In fact, anion exchange chromatography is a priori undesirable as an initial step for large-scale antibody purification, since virtually all of the proteins and dyes are bound, which drastically reduces the capacity of the matrix available to bind immunoglobulin (9-12,24). This reduction in capacity is a particular disadvantage when one is developing a method, since analytical chromatography on these matrices often does not correctly predict the chromatographic profile in the presence of the overloaded conditions typically used for scale-up to preparative chromatography (9-12,20-22,24). With very few exceptions (9-11), totally different surface chemistries must be used if preparative chromatography on traditional low-pressure, open columns is to be scaled-up from methods development conducted on analytical HPLC media.

B. Affinity Chromatography

Another method for antibody purification that has recently gained wide acceptance is the use of protein A (for IgG), Jacalin (for IgA), antiimmuno-globulin, specific antigen, and other affinity matrices (1,13,25,26). The development of these materials represents a major breakthrough in the field of antibody purification, since in many cases the monoclonal of interest may be separated in a highly purified state with minimal contamination (9,13,25,26). Protein A and antigen- or antibody-based affinity matrices usually require harsh elution conditions (25,26) that may denature the monoclonal antibody and reduce immunologic activity or bind immunoglobulins irreversibly. Another drawback of protein A is its inability to bind all antibody classes and subclasses, as well as antibody fragments, antibody conjugates, hybrids, and chemically modified immunoglobulins (9,13,25,26). In addition, protein A or affinity matrices have a low capacity, short column lifetime, and high cost, and as such are uneconomical for preparative or process-scale purifications.

C. Hydroxyapatite Chromatography

Hydroxyapatite is a useful chromatographic matrix for the purification of monoclonal antibodies (13). Its major advantage over conventional non-affinity methods is that most antibodies appear to be bound more strongly than the majority of the other common protein contaminants. However, hydroxyapatite is fragile, produces high back pressures and low flow rates, tends to bind immunoglobulin nonspecifically and irreversibly, requires long chromatographic run times, and suffers from extremely short column lifetime (9,13,27). The capacity of hydroxyapatite is up to 15 times lower than that on chromatographic materials based on silica or even organic resins (9-11). These problems, along with broad peaks, produce a purified antibody preparation that is substantially diluted.

As a result of many of the disadvantages inherent to these separation techniques, protein chemists have been forced to use a series of elaborate purification steps to achieve the desired level of antibody purity. For protein chemists or process engineers faced with the task of purifying numerous antibodies from a number of sources, the most practical approach would involve one or two high resolving chromatographic matrices having universal applicability with minor adjustments in purification protocols to enable the attainment of any desired level of purity at any level from analytical to scale-up.

IV. ABx–ANTIBODY EXCHANGER

The requirements for an economical chromatographic matrix that could rapidly purify large quantities of antibodies to homogeneity compelled us to investigate synthetic approaches to construct a chromatographic surface that would bind antibodies more selectively than conventional ion exchange matrices. Chemists at J. T. Baker developed the ABx^{TM} (antibody exchanger) matrix that uses "mixed mode" interactions as the basis, silica gel as the most advantageous support, and a proprietary hydrophilic polymeric coverage to increase stability, eliminate nonspecific protein binding, and maximize recovery. This chromatographic matrix behaves like an ion exchanger in that immunoglobulins are resolved via the manipulation of buffer species, pH, and ionic strength. However, it also exhibits an affinity-like sensitivity towards all immunoglobulins indicative of more subtle, more complex interactions.

The major advantage of ABx is that is binds mostly antibodies while exhibiting little or no affinity for albumins, transferrins, proteases, or pH indicator dyes from tissue culture media (Table 1). Therefore, ABx can be used as a rapid fractionation medium to remove selectively nonpyrogenic immunoglobulins of any class or type from ascites fluids, serum-based cell culture media, or serum/plasma of any species. The purity of the immunoglobulin obtained in a single purification step on ABx varies from about 70 to 99+%.

Table 1   Retention Times of Polyclonal and Monoclonal Immunoglobulins on BAKERBOND^{TM} ABx[a]

Source	Antibody or protein	Antigen if known	Retention time (min)
Mouse ascites	$IgG_{1,k}$		36
Mouse ascites	$IgG_{2a,k}$		26

Table 1   (Continued)

Source	Antibody or protein	Antigen if known	Retention time (min)
Mouse ascites	$IgG_{2a,k}$		26
Mouse ascites	$IgG_{2b,k}$		26
Mouse ascites	$IgG_{2b,k}$		26
Mouse ascites	IgG_3		30
Mouse ascites	IgA		16
Mouse ascites	IgA		25
Mouse ascites	IgM		28
Mouse ascites	IgG	BSA	29
Mouse ascites	IgG	SRBC	40
Mouse ascites	IgG		35
Mouse ascites	IgG		45
Mouse ascites	IgG		22
Mouse ascites	IgD		40
Mouse ascites	IgG		60/67
Mouse ascites	IgG	HCG	25
Mouse ascites	IgG	HCG	27
Mouse ascites	IgG	HCG	27
Mouse ascites	IgM		52/60
Mouse ascites	IgM		60
Mouse ascites	IgM		68
Mouse ascites	IgM		68
Mouse ascites	IgG		30
Mouse ascites	IgG	I1–2	42
Tissue culture	IgG	I1–2	42
Tissue culture	IgG	Int	40
Tissue culture	IgG	Ren	31
Tissue culture	IgG		45
Tissue culture	IgG		50
Tissue culture	IgM		30

Table 1   (Continued)

Source	Antibody or protein	Antigen if known	Retention time (min)
Tissue culture	IgM	ODC	27
Tissue culture	IgG		30
Human serum	IgG	(polyclonal)	22–35
Human serum	IgG	(polyclonal)	22–31
Bovine serum	IgG	(polyclonal)	22–31
Guinea pig serum	IgG	(polyclonal)	22–31
Mouse serum	IgG	(polyclonal)	25–37
Rabbit serum	IgG	(polyclonal)	24–32
Bovine serum	Albumin		3
Human serum	Albumin		3
Mouse serum	Albumin		3
Bovine serum	Transferrin		3
Human serum	Transferrin		3
Mouse serum	Transferrin		3
Various	Proteases		3

[a]All retention times were determined on a BAKERBOND ABx analytical column (4.6 × 250 mm). 250 μl of sample was chromatographed over a 60 min linear gradient of 10 mM MES, pH 6.0 to 250 mM KH_2PO_4, pH 6.8, with a flow rate of 1.0 ml/min.

V. GENERAL PROPERTIES OF ABx

ABx media are made from high-quality, closely sized chromatographic silica that produce high-column efficiencies and high resolution (Tables 1 and 2, Fig. 1). This silica base is derivatized with a proprietary hydrophilic polymeric backbone that serves three purposes: (1) it covers up nonspecific interaction sites on the silica surface, leading to quantitative recovery of antibody mass and immunological activity; (2) it "protects" the entire surface of the silica base, thereby increasing chemical and physical stability, and column lifetime; and (3) it increases ligand density and the capacity of the matrix to bind immunoglobulins (Table 2; Appendix 3, Section VI).

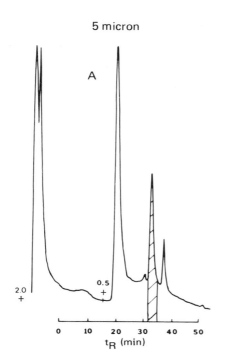

Figure 1 Chromatographic profile of the same cell culture supernatant
chromatographed on 5 μm ABx, 15 μm ABx, and 40 μm BAKERBOND ABx.
Chromatography was conducted on stainless steel HPLC column (7.75 ✕
100 mm) containing 5, 15, or 40 μm BAKERBOND ABx. The mobile phase
consisted of an initial (A) buffer of 10 mM MES, pH 5.6, and a final (B)
buffer of 1 M NaOAc, pH 7.0, with a linear gradient (100% A–100% B) over
1 hr. The flow rate was 1.0 ml/min and this produced back-pressures of 200,
15, and 3 psi for the 5, 15, and 40 μm (PREPSCALE) particles, respectively.
In each case, 0.3 ml of a 20-fold concentrated tissue culture media ultrafiltrate (diluted to 1.2 ml with buffer A) was loaded onto the column. The
void volume peak was composed of albumins, transferrins, proteases, and
phenol red, and the cross-hatched peak contained the immunoglobulin. The
proteins were detected by ultraviolet absorbance at 280 nm and the attenua-
tion (absorbance units full scale, AUFS) was decreased from 2.0 to 0.5
following the elution of the void volume peak as indicated (+) in each
chromatogram (to visualize better the antibody peak).

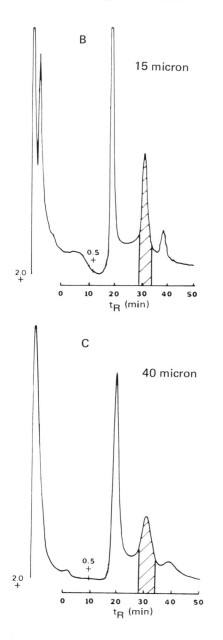

Table 2 BAKERBOND ABx and MAb^{TM}: General Properties

Matrix	Average silica particle size (μm)	Particle shape	Pore size (Å)	Typical back-pressures[a] (psi) A	B	Approximate capacity[b]	Stability (pH range)
ABx	5	Spherical	300	200	1,000	0.4 mEq/g[c]	2–10
ABx	15	Spheroidal	300	15	80	0.7 mEq/g	2–10
ABx	40	Irregular	275	3	30	1.0 mEq/g	2–10
MAb	5	Spherical	300	200	1,000	0.7 mEq/g[c]	2–10
MAb	15	Spheroidal	300	15	80	0.8 mEq/g	2–10
MAb	40	Irregular	275	3	30	2.0 mEq/g	2–10

[a]At a flow rate of 1.0 ml/min with (A) 7.75 × 100 mm or (B) 4.6 × 250 mm columns.
[b]Ion exchange groups and mgIgG bound/g packing.
[c]150 mg IgG/g ABx.
[d]See Figure 1.

VI. USES OF ABx

The selectivity and resolving power of the ABx surface chemistry, plus the rigid, polymer-coated silica support with its high ligand density and high capacity, make ABx a versatile tool for analysis and purification.

A. Analysis, Characterization, and Production Monitoring

Traditionally, the analysis of supernatants from large-scale fermentations as well as hybridoma selection and screening processes have been conducted with by sodium dodecyl sulfate polyacrylamide gel electrophoresis (SDS PAGE), affinity chromatography, immunologic methods, amino acid analysis, gel filtration chromatography, and ion exchange chromatography (9–14,28,29). All these methods tend to be rather slow, give semiquantitative results, and/or require sophisticated apparatus and techniques. Trace levels of monoclonal antibodies in complex mixtures can be chromatographed on ABx for hybridoma subcloning, antibody characterization, process monitoring, optimization of harvest time, tracking genetic drift, and purification monitoring (Appendix, Sections C and D). Alternatively, if accuracy is less critical, solid phase extraction of monoclonals with ABx spe^{TM} columns facilitates the rapid spectrophotometric analysis and/or the simultaneous clean-up of numerous samples (Appendix 3, Section IV, Fig. 2).

Mass recovery (%)	Proteins bound	Exchange mechanism	Typical efficiency (plates/m)	Relative resolution	Stability (hr of use)
>97	Immunoglobulins	"Mixed mode"	50,000	Highest	>1,000
>97	Immunoglobulins	"Mixed mode"	6,000	High	>1,000
>97	Immunoglobulins	"Mixed mode"	2,000	Lower[d]	>1,000
>97	Most proteins	Anion	50,000	Highest	>1,000
>97	Most proteins	Anion	6,000	High	>1,000
>97	Most proteins	Anion	2,000	Lower	>1,000

B. Purification

1. Method Development for Scale-Up

To facilitate method development for the scale-up to low-pressure preparative antibody purification, the ABx surface chemistry has been bonded to three silica sizes that produce bonded phases with remarkably similar chromatographic properties (Fig. 1, Table 1). These silica sizes include 5 μm spherical silica for analytical high-performance column chromatography (HPLC) or for a high-resolution, high-purity final step purification; 15 μm spheroidal silica for high resolution, low to medium pressure analytical or preparative chromatography; and economical 40 μm (BAKERBOND PREPSCALE) irregularly shaped "bulk" silica for large-scale batch or solid-phase extraction and traditional low-pressure, open-column chromatography. The differences in resolution on these three particle sizes are minimized due to the similar surface chemistry used in each case. Method development is more rapid on 5 or 15 μm ABx since resolution, purity, and specific activities are high, while elution volumes and buffer requirements are low (facilitating analysis, assay, and identification).

2. Preparative Column Chromatography

Since the majority of proteins are not bound by ABx, the relative capacity to bind antibody (150 mg/g ABx) is significantly enhanced. In a typical

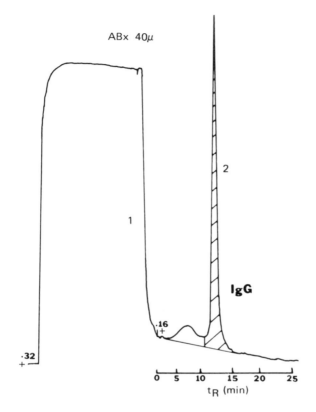

Figure 2 Semipreparative chromatography of serum-based cell culture supernatant on 40 μm BAKERBOND PREPSCALE ABx. 1.5 L cell culture media
was concentrated 20-fold by ultrafiltration, diluted five-fold with buffer A,
and chromatographed on a column (21.2 × 150 mm) containing 15 g 40 μm
PREPSCALE ABx. The mobile phase consisted of (A) an initial buffer of
10 mM MES, pH 5.6, and (B) a final buffer of 250 mM KH_2PO_4, pH 6.8.
The gradient was linear (100% A–100% B) over 40 min. The flow rate was
20 ml/min and the back-pressure was 20 psi. The detector (UV at 280 nm)
sensitivity was increased from 0.32 to 0.16 AUFS following the elution of
the "void volume" peak (1) that contained the nonbound proteins (albumins,
transferrins, proteases, etc.). Peak (2) contained greater than 95% of the
original IgG at a purity greater than 90% by SDS PAGE (cross-hatched area).

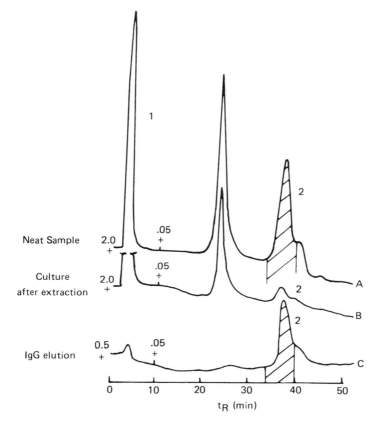

Neat Sample

Culture
after extraction

IgG elution

t_R (min)

(A)

Figure 3 BAKERBOND ABx batch extractions of monoclonal antibodies from two cell culture supernatants as monitored by ABx (5 μm) HPLC column chromatography. Analytical conditions for the ABx chromatographic monitoring are the same as in Figure 1 except that buffer B consisted of 125 mM KH_2PO_4, pH 6.8 and the column size was 4.6 × 250 mm. Peak 1 contains the albumins and transferrins, peak 2 is the monoclonal antibody. Note the low levels of antibody being selectively removed by ABx and the increase in recorder sensitivity on the chromatograms following the elution of the unbound proteins, (+). Following the extraction procedure, the IgG purity was 85% by SDS PAGE analysis.

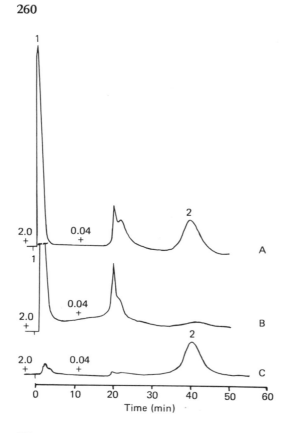

(B)

Figure 3   (Continued)

semipreparative separation, a small column dry-packed with approximately 15 g
40 μm BAKERBOND PREPSCALE ABx was used to purify over 100 mg IgG
from 1.5 L serum-based cell culture media, with quantitative recovery of
highly purified monoclonal (Fig. 2; analytical runs; see Fig. 1).

3. Batch Extraction With ABx

One of the oldest yet simplest methods to purify proteins is by "batch"
extraction. The method is quick, easy, and economical and requires no
column, pumps, or other chromatographic equipment. The protein of interest
is "selectively" removed from crude biological mixtures by adding a given
separation ("chromatographic") media or absorbent (Appendix 3, Section III).

The ABx matrix operates similarly to an affinity-like adsorbent towards immunoglobulins by selectively removing antibodies from ascites fluid, cell culture media, or serum/plasma (Fig. 3). While soft gels contain fines and require centrifugation or long periods of time to settle by gravity, the 40 μm BAKERBOND PREPSCALE ABx separates from the aqueous phase within minutes. ABx is easily sterilized and regenerated, and does not support microbial growth (Appendix 3, Section I), making batch extractions with ABx suitable for large-scale applications where aseptic conditions and extreme product purity are required. The exact conditions required for aqueous batch extraction of proteins on ABx media (Appendix 3, Section III), as well as the kinetics of the process may be conveniently monitored and maximized using ABx analytical HPLC columns (Fig. 3).

VII. ABx VERSUS ANION EXCHANGERS

The high degree of resolution achieved on the ABx is illustrated when a series of collected fractions from the ABx are rechromatographed on a high-performance anion exchanger such as the MAb (Fig. 4). While greater than 90% of the proteins present within serum-supplemented tissue culture media is not bound by ABx, these proteins are bound by anion exchangers. In fact, rechromatography of the ABx void volume fraction (which contains these nonbound proteins) on an anion exchanger produces a chromatographic profile virtually identical to that of the neat sample itself (Fig. 4). A substantial portion of contaminating proteins coelute with the monoclonal antibody on high-performance anion exchangers. These are totally resolved from the immunoglobulins on the ABx.

VIII. EFFECTS OF BUFFERS ON ELUTION PROFILE

Another major advantage of ABx over other chromatographic matrices is the dramatic changes in elution profile and final product purity that occur when various buffer systems are used as the mobile phase. Any given protein has numerous different sites at which physical interactions may occur. Bonded phases such as the ABx, which consist of "mixed modes" of interacting groups (multiple ligand types), offer several types of absorbtion mechanisms and binding affinities/types. Due to the differences in buffering capacity, pH, ionic strength, and ion composition of various buffers (Appendix 3, Sections 7 and 8) the physical interactions between any given protein and the ABx chromatographic matrix may differ substantially. As a result, dramatic changes in selectivity and resolution have been achieved by manipulating buffer conditions to optimize resolution in a one-step purification scheme (Fig. 5).

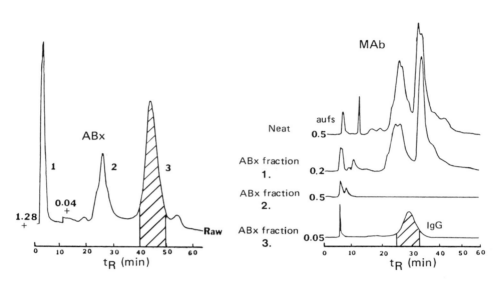

Figure 4   Rechromatography of ABx fractions of a serum-based cell culture
medium on a high-performance anion exchange matrix (BAKERBOND MAb).
Neat hybridoma tissue culture media (0.3 ml) was chromatographed on a
40 μm PREPSCALE ABx column, and the three major ABx peaks (1, 2, 3)
were rechromatographed on a 15 μm MAb column. More than 95% of the
total protein was not bound by the ABx (fraction 1), while these nonimmunoglobulin proteins were bound and even coeluted with the monoclonal antibody
on the MAb and other anion exchangers. The purity of the monoclonal
fraction (3) from the ABx column was greater than 90% IgG by SDS PAGE.
Note the changes in recorder sensitivity (AUFS; +) and the low levels of
monoclonal present. Analytical conditions for the ABx chromatogram were
the same as those in Figure 1 except that the elution buffer was 125 mM
KH_2PO_4, pH 6.0, and the column size was 4.6 × 250 mm. Peak 1 consisted
of the albumins, transferrins, proteases, and phenol red, and peak 3 contained
the monoclonal antibody (cross-hatched area). Anion exchange chromatography
was conducted on an HPLC column (4.6 × 250 mm) packed with 15 μm
BAKERBOND MAb matrix. The mobile phase for the MAb consisted of
(A) an initial buffer of 10 mM KH_2PO_4, pH 6.6, and (B) a final buffer of
500 mM KH_2PO_4, pH 6.6, with a linear gradient (100% A–50% B) over 1 hr.
The flow rate was 1.0 ml/min with a back-pressure of 150 psi, with ultraviolet (280 nm) detection at various AUFS (+).

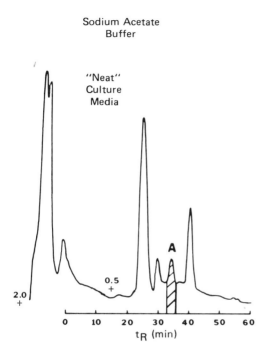

Figure 5 Effects of buffer conditions on the elution profile and purification of a monoclonal antibody present at low levels in a serum-based cell culture supernatant. A high level of purity (peaks A and B are greater than 85% IgG) was achieved in a single step with either elution buffer system (sodium acetate or ammonium sulfate), despite the low level of monoclonal antibody present (less than 1% of the total protein). Rechromatography of peak A in the presence of ammonium sulfate buffer produced homogeneous antibody (peak C) as determined by SDS PAGE. Chromatography was conducted on BAKERBOND GOLD HPLC columns (7.75 × 100 mm) packed with 5 μm ABx. The mobile phases consisted of (A) an initial buffer of 10 mM MES, pH 5.6, and a (B) final buffer of either 500 mM NaOAc, pH 7.0 (as in chromatogram A, above left), or 250 mM $(NH_4)_2SO_4$ plus 10 mM NaOAc, pH 5.6 (as in chromatograms B, above right, and C in the insert). The gradient was linear (100% A–100% B) over 1.5 hr and the flow rate was 0.7 ml/min with a back-pressure of 150 psi. The sample load was 0.4 ml neat medium (diluted to 1.2 ml with A buffer). The detection was by ultraviolet light at 280 nm with the sensitivity changed from 2.0 to 0.5 AUFS following the elution of the void volume peak (+).

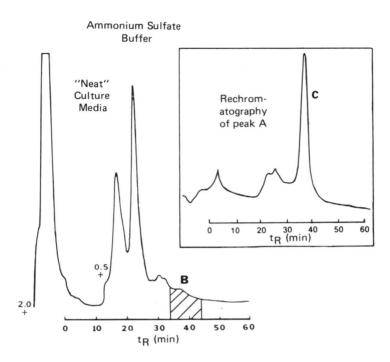

Figure 5   (Continued)

Furthermore, rechromatographing the immunoglobulin-containing peak under
a second set of buffer conditions typically produces homogeneous antibody
(Fig. 5). Initial results indicate that KH_2PO_4, $(NH_4)_2SO_4$, NaCl, and NaOAc
buffer systems each give totally distinct elution profiles (Appendix 3,
Section 8).

In the presence of ammonium sulfate buffer, immunoglobulins are bound
by ABx more strongly than any other proteins present in mouse ascites fluid,
plasma, fetal bovine serum, or serum-based hybridoma tissue culture media
(results not shown). This is a particular advantage in the "preparative mode."
Rather than hindering resolution, column overload actually tends to increase
resolution by virtue of displacement chromatography of contaminating proteins bound to ABx less tightly than the antibody. This phenomenon also
occurs with other buffer systems. The resolution was not reduced on a preparative column (Fig. 2) on which approximately 20 times more tissue
culture ultrafiltrate was loaded per gram of resin than on the comparable
analytical column (Fig. 1).

IX. RESOLUTION OF ANTIBODY SPECIES

Under similar chromatographic conditions, antibodies have been found to elute from ABx at a wide range of retention times (Table 1). Variations in elution times ranging from 16 to 68 min are apparently the result of subtle difference in antibody structure and molecular diversity that are as yet not totally defined.

Whereas the variability in antibody elution times may be a disadvantage on anion exchangers due to possible coelution of the antibody with albumin or transferrin, it represents a distinct advantage of ABx. It facilitates the resolution of different monoclonals with minimal possibility of contamination by the unbound, nonimmunoglobulin proteins. ABx is capable of fractionating the heterogeneous population of polyclonal antibodies present within serum/plasma (Fig. 6). ABx is also able to separate monoclonal antibody from "host" (serum polyclonal) immunoglobulin contaminants in mouse ascites fluid (Fig. 7). Likewise, ABx is capable of high resolution of multiple antibody species secreted from "double-producing" hybridomas (Figs. 8 and 9). Multiple forms of IgGs and IgMs have been separated in a highly purified state from ascites fluids and cell culture media, respectively, with minimal method development (Fig. 8). Multiple forms of myeloma IgG_1 and monoclonal IgG_{2a} from a single hybridoma have also been resolved on ABx with either gradient elution or isocratic elution (Fig. 9). Such a technique will no doubt facilitate basic research and development in the field of immunology (15), as well as the purification of truly homogeneous antibody preparations.

X. TWO-DIMENSIONAL CHROMATOGRAPHY: ABx AND MAb

Although many antibodies elute from ABx as electrophoretically pure peaks, the immunoglobulin fractions that contain minor contaminants may yield homogeneous antibody by direct chromatography on a high-performance anion exchange matrix such as the MAb (9–11,19,20). The mechanisms of separation on these two complementary bonded phases are entirely different. Together MAb and ABx offer selectivity and resolution that are greatly enhanced relative to any single chromatographic medium alone.

An example of two-dimensional chromatography using ABx-bonded phase followed by MAb-bonded phase was carried out with a sample of cell culture supernatant and with human plasma (Figs. 10 and 11). The technique involves collecting the immunoglobulin-containing peak from the ABx column, diluting with two or three parts distilled water or MAb starting buffer, and reinjecting this lower level of protein onto a smaller MAb column. The method can be applied on an analytical or preparative scale to purify virtually any immunoglobulin to homogeneity.

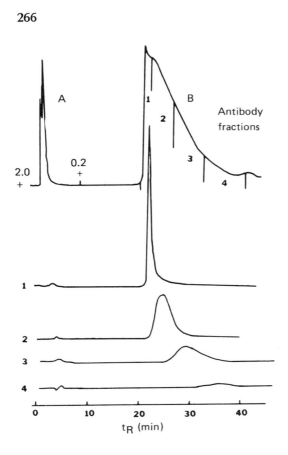

Figure 6 Fractionation of the diverse antibody species present in human plasma on 40 μm PREPSCALE ABx. Neat human plasma was chromatographed on 40 μm PREPSCALE ABx and the antibody-containing fractions (1, 2, 3, and 4) were collected and rechromatographed under identical conditions. Polyclonal antibodies may be "fractionated" on ABx due to their polydisperse nature, and further "fractionation" may be achieved by rechromatography in the presence of a second or third buffer system (data not shown). Analytical conditions were the same as in Figure 1 except that the column size was 4.6 × 250 mm and the final (B) buffer was 125 mM KH_2PO_4, pH 5.6.

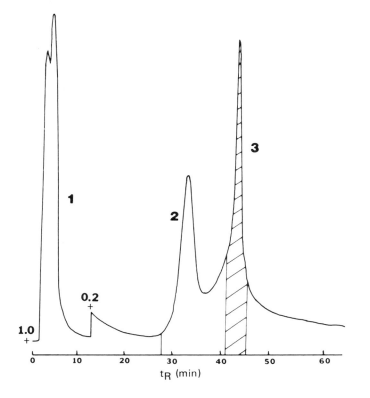

Figure 7 Separation of contaminating "host" (mouse serum polyclonal) antibodies from a monoclonal antibody present in mouse ascites fluid on 15 μm BAKERBOND ABx. Analytical conditions were the same as those given in Figure 1, except that the column size was 4.6 × 250 mm and buffer A was 10 mM KH_2PO_4, pH 6.0, and buffer B was 125 mM KH_2PO_4, pH 6.8. The sample load was 0.4 ml neat sample (diluted to 1.2 ml with A buffer). Peak 1 consisted of albumin, transferrin, and proteases; peak 2 was the "host" IgG, and peak 3 was the monoclonal antibody.

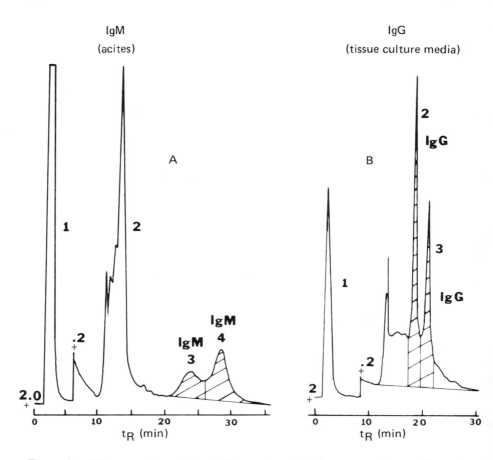

Figure 8 ABx separation of two IgMs produced in the same mouse ascites fluid or two IgGs produced by the same hybridoma grown in culture. Analytical conditions were the same as in Figure 1 except that the column size was 4.6 × 250 mm and buffer B was 500 mM KH$_2$PO$_4$, pH 6.8. A. Peak 1 consisted of albumin, transferrin, and proteases; peak 2 contained weakly bound proteins; and peaks 3 and 4 (cross-hatched areas) were two distinct IgM species both greater than 95% pure by SDS PAGE. B. Analytical conditions were the same as in Figure 1 except that the column size was 4.6 × 250 mm and the starting (A) buffer was 10 mM MES, pH 6.0, buffer B was 250 mM KH$_2$PO$_4$, pH 5.6, and a "step" gradient was used (100% A for 10 min, then step to 20% B followed by a linear gradient from 20% B to 50% B over 60 min). In each case, 0.5 ml neat sample (diluted to 1.5 ml with buffer A) was injected. Peaks 2 and 3 (cross-hatched areas) are both IgGs at greater than 95% purity by SDS PAGE.

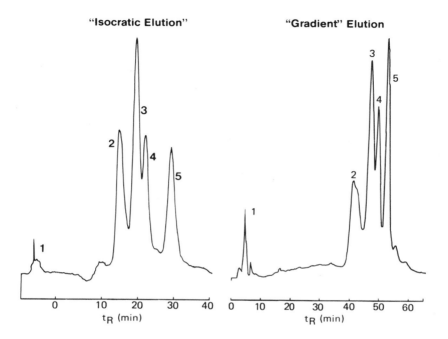

Figure 9   ABx chromatographic profile of a "monoclonal antibody" purified from a serum-free media by ultrafiltration and two chromatographic steps on a high-performance anion exchange matrix. Although the purified antibody(ies) eluted as a single peak on the anion exchanger, ABx was able to resolve small amounts of albumin and transferrin contamination (peak 1) and multiple forms of immunoglobulin (peaks 2, 3, 4, and 5). Immunologic methods later revealed the presence of both myeloma IgG_1 (65% of the total IgG) and monoclonal IgG_{2a} (35% of the total IgG). The fact that different ABx chromatographic profiles were obtained with different elution buffers (data not shown) further suggests that ABx may be valuable in purifying individual immunoglobulins to total homogeneity. Analytical conditions are the same as in Figure 1 except that in the "isocratic" run a longer (4.6 X 250 mm) column was used; after equilibrating the column in the initial buffer (100% A), a step gradient to 25% final (B) buffer was used and the antibodies were eluted isocratically.

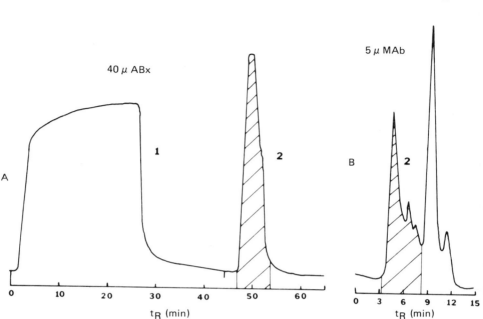

Figure 10 Sequential purification of human polyclonal antibodies from human plasma on ABx and MAb. Neat human plasma was fractionated on 40 μm PREPSCALE ABx and the peak (2) containing the IgG was diluted twice and rechromatographed on a 5 μm MAb column to achieve higher immunoglobulin purity. Analytical conditions for ABx were the same as in Figure 1 except that 8 g protein were loaded onto a 21.1 × 150 mm column of 40 μm PREPSCALE ABx with a flow rate of 20 ml/min and buffer B was 250 mM KH_2PO_4, pH 6.8. Analytical conditions for anion exchange chromatography on MAb are given in Figure 4 with peak 2 being greater than 95% pure IgG by SDS PAGE analysis.

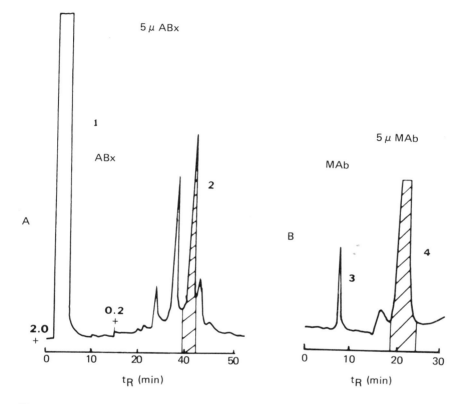

Figure 11   Sequential purification of monoclonal antibody from a cell culture supernatant on ABx and MAb. Neat hybridoma tissue culture media (0.5 ml ultrafiltrate diluted to 1.5 ml with A buffer) was chromatographed on ABx and the peak containing the monoclonal antibody was diluted twice and rechromatographed on an MAb column to give homogeneous IgG. Analytical conditions for the ABx chromatogram are the same as those given in Figure 1 except that the initial (A) buffer was 10 mM MES, pH 6.0, and buffer B was 125 mM KH_2PO_4, pH 6.8. Analytical conditions for the MAb run were the same as in Figure 4 except that the final (B) buffer was 250 mM KH_2PO_4, pH 6.5. Peak 1 was composed of albumins and transferrins, peak 2 was IgG (80–90% pure) plus impurities (see peak 3), and peak 4 was homogeneous IgG (by SDS PAGE analysis).

XI. SUMMARY

By virtue of its ability to bind immunoglobulins rather selectively, ABx is similar to protein A. However, it differs from protein A in a number of important respects. Unlike protein A, ABx is able to bind all antibodies (IgG_1, IgG_{2a}, IgG_{2b}, IgG_3, IgA, IgD, IgE, and IgM) as well as antibody hybrids, bispecific hybrids, antibody–protein conjugates, and chemically modified antibodies (9–11). In contrast to affinity matrices, antibodies are eluted from ABx in small volumes of buffer at physiological pH and ionic strength with quantitative recovery of mass (Table 2) and immunologic activity (results not shown). Furthermore, the susceptibility of protein-based chromatographic media to biodegradation, proteolytic digestion, and ligand or endotoxin leakage make chemically defined matrices such as ABx an attractive alternative (Appendix 3, Section I).

ABx has a capacity to bind immunoglobulins (Table 2) approximately 15 times higher than that of protein A or hydroxyapatite (9–11,13). ABx is also more "rugged" and durable than hydroxyapatite or affinity matrices, and has been used for up to 1,000 hr with little loss in resolution or capacity. These advantages, along with the ability to use higher flow rates at lower back pressures (9–11,13), allow for substantially higher throughputs for more economical operation.

In any protein purification problem, several factors are of utmost importance: high column capacity, resolution, recovery, and specificity; ease of use; regeneration and sterilization; speed; throughput; durability; longevity; versatility of use; and economy. The ABx-bonded phase has been designed with each of these in mind.

As new types of monoclonal antibodies are purified and as purity requirements increase, it becomes increasingly apparent that the molecular diversity inherent in the immunoglobulin family makes a universal single-step purification method less likely. However, the development of dedicated chromatographic matrices such as the ABx, which utilize composite surface interactions to maximize selective antibody binding and resolution, represents a major step in the right direction.

ACKNOWLEDGMENTS

The author acknowledges the assistance of Dr. Laura Jane Crane and Dr. Sally Seaver for helpful discussions with the preparation of this text, Dr. Michael P. Henry for his assistance with the batch extractions, Dr. Steve Berkowitz for the two-dimensional chromatography of human plasma, Mrs. Joyce G. Guenther for her work on the solid phase extraction with ABx, Mrs. Diane Rush for SDS PAGE analysis, and particularly Dr. Hugh E. Ramsden and

Mr. Joseph Horvath for their eloquent synthesis and help in optimizing the ABx surface chemistry.

REFERENCES

1. Kohler, G. and Milstein, C. (1975). Continuous cultures of fused cells secreting antibody of predefined specificity. *Nature 256*: 495–497.
2. Yelton, D. E. and Scharff, M. D. (1981). Monoclonal antibodies: A powerful new tool in biology and medicine. *Annu. Rev. Biochem. 50*: 657–680.
3. Ritz, J. and Schlossman, S. F. (1982). Utilization of monoclonal antibodies in the treatment of leukemia and lymphoma. *Blood 59*: 1–11.
4. Larson, S. M., Brown, J. P., Wright, P. W., Carasquillo, J. A., Hellstrom, I., and Hellstrom, K. E. (1983). Imaging of melanoma and I^{131}-labeled monoclonal antibodies. *J. Nucl. Med. 24*: 123–129.
5. Staehelin, T., Hobbs, D. S., Kung, H.-F., Lai, C.-Y., and Pestka, S. (1981). Purification and characterization of recombinant human leukocyte interferon (IFLrA) with monoclonal antibodies. *J. Biol. Chem. 256*: 9750–9754.
6. Calton, G. J. (1984). Immunosorbent separations. *Methods Enzymol. 104*: 381–387.
7. Shimizu, F., Wang, R., and Varga, M. (1983). Growth hormone quantitation in human serum using monoclonal antibodies to a two-site IRMA. *Clin. Chem. 29*: 1245–1250.
8. Wang, R., Bermudez, W. F., Saunders, R. L., Present, W. A., Bartholomew, R. M., and Adams, T. (1981). The TANDEM^{TM} PAP system: A simplified radioimmunometric assay employing monoclonal antibodies to prostatic acid phosphatase. *Clin. Chem. 27*: 1063–1069.
9. Nau, D. R., Berkowtiz, S. A., Henry, M. P., and Crane, L. J. (1986). A multidimensional approach to monoclonal antibody purification. Poster H-13 presented at the Fifth Annual Congress for Hybridoma Research, Baltimore, Maryland, January 26–29.
10. Nau, D. R., Henry, M. P., Berkowitz, S. A., Crane, L. J., Ramsden, H. E., Guenther, J. G., and Zief, M. (1986). Monoclonal antibody purification by solid phase extraction. Poster H-14 presented at the Fifth Annual Congress for Hybridoma Research, Baltimore, Maryland, January 26–29.
11. Nau, D. R., Henry, M. P., Berkowitz, S. A., and Crane, L. J. (1986). Determination of monoclonal antibody concentrations by HPLC. Poster H-15 presented at the Fifth Annual Congress for Hybridoma Research, Baltimore, Maryland, January 26–29.
12. Gemski, M. J., Doctor, B. P., Gentry, J. K., Pluskal, M. J., and Strickler, M. P. (1985). Single step purification of monoclonal antibody from murine ascites and tissue culture fluids by anion exchange high performance liquid chromatography. *BioTechniques 3*: 378–384.

13. Brooks, T. L. and Stevens, A. (1985). Techniques for purifying mono-
    clonal antibodies. *Am. Lab.*, pp. 54–64.
14. Bailon, P., Drugazima, N., and Nishikawa, A. H. (1986). Large scale purifi-
    cation of monoclonal antibodies from intracapsular supernatants and
    ascites fluids. Paper 210, presented at Biotechnology '86, New Orleans,
    LA, January 29–30.
15. Duberstein, R. (1986). Scientists develop new technique for producing
    biospecific monoclonals. *Genetic Engin. News*, pp. 22–25.
16. Levy, H. B. and Sober, H. A. (1960). A simple chromatographic method
    for preparation of gamma-globulin. *Proc. Soc. Exp. Biol. Med. 103*: 250.
17. Garvey, J. S., Cremer, N. E., and Susodorf, D. H. (1977). A laboratory
    text for instruction and research. In *Methods in Immunology*, Reading,
    MA, Addison-Wesley, pp. 223–226.
18. Fahey, J. L. and Terry, E. W. (1978). *Handbook of Experimental Im-
    munology.* Edited by D. M. Weir. London, Blackwell, *1*: 8.1–8.16.
19. Flashner, M. and Henry, M. P. (1984). Production-scale purification of
    monoclonal antibodies by high performance ion exchange chromatography.
    Paper 811, presented at the Fourth International Symposium on HPLC of
    Proteins, Peptides, and Polynucleotides, Baltimore, Maryland, December
    10–12.
20. Berkowitz, S. A., Crane, L. J., Guenther, J. G., Henry, M. P., Nau, D. R.,
    and Ramsden, H. E. (1985). A multidimensional approach to the problem
    of molecular diversity in monoclonal antibody purification. Paper 1002,
    presented at the Fifth International Symposium on HPLC of Proteins,
    Polypeptides, and Polynucleotides, Toronto, Canada, November 4–6.
21. Deschamps, J. R., Kildreth, J. E. K., Derr, D., and August, J. T. (1985).
    A high performance liquid chromatographic procedure for the purification
    of mouse monoclonal antibodies. *Anal. Biochem. 147*: 451–454.
22. Clezardin, P., McGregor, J. L., Manach, M., Bonkerche, H., and Deschavanne,
    M. (1985). One-step procedure for the rapid isolation of mouse mono-
    clonal antibodies and their antigen binding fragments by fast protein liquid
    chromatography on a Mono-Q anion exchange column. *J. Chromatogr.
    319*: 67–77.
23. Burchiel, S. W., Billman, J. R., and Alber, T. R. (1984). Rapid and efficient
    purification of mouse monoclonal antibodies from ascites fluid using high
    performance liquid chromatography. *J. Immunol. Methods 69*: 33–44.
24. Nazareth, A. (1985). Personal communication; Stephen DiScullio, per-
    sonal communication with the author; personal observation.
25. Ey, P. L., Prowse, S. J., and Jenkin, C. R. (1978). Isolation of pure IgG_1,
    IgG_{2a}, IgG_{2b} immunoglobulins from mouse serum using protein A
    Sepharose. *Immunochemistry 15*: 429–436.
26. Wofsy, L. and Burr, B. (1969). A use of affinity chromatography for the
    specific purification of antibodies and antigens. *J. Immunol. 103*: 380–
    383.

27. Hirano, H., Nishimura, T., and Iwamura, T. (1985). High flow rate hydro-
     xyapatites. *Anal. Biochem. 150*: 228–234.
28. Colonick, S. P., Kaplan, N. O., Langone, J. J., and Van Vunakis, H. (eds.)
     (1981). Immunochemical techniques (Part B). *Methods Enzymol. 73*:
     21–34.
29. Frej, A.-K., Gustafsson, J.-G., and Hedman, P. (1984). FPLC for monitor-
     ing microbial and mammalian cell cultures. *Biotechnology 2*: 777–781.

14

High-Performance Liquid Chromatography Characterization and Purification of Monoclonal Antibodies

HECTOR JUAREZ–SALINAS, TIMOTHY L. BROOKS, and GARY S. OTT*
Bio-Rad Laboratories, Richmond, California

ROBERT E. PETERS†
University of California at San Diego, San Diego, California

LARRY STANKER
Lawrence Livermore National Laboratory, Livermore, California

I. INTRODUCTION

Since their discovery (1), monoclonal antibodies have found a wide range of research and industrial applications. As the number of applications grow, the need for fast and automated high-resolution purification procedures for monoclonal antibodies has become apparent. As shown in this chapter, high performance liquid chromatography (HPLC) is ideally fitted to fulfill this requirement. The chapter is divided into two main sections: the first is devoted to sample characterization and determination of antibody class and concentration using size exclusion HPLC (SE-HPLC). The second section deals with the issue of monoclonal antibody purification and provides the rationale for the use of protein A HPLC (PA-HPLC) and high performance hydroxylapatite (HPHT). Appendix 5 describes the materials and sample preparation protocols used in these procedures.

Present affiliation: Chiron Corporation, Emeryville, California.
†*Present affiliation*: Cytotech Inc., San Diego, California.

II. CHARACTERIZATION OF MONOCLONAL ANTIBODIES

A. Size Exclusion High Performance Liquid Chromatography

Before starting the purification, it is necessary to obtain information on the class and concentration of the monoclonal antibody present in the sample. Likewise, it is also necessary to monitor the efficiency of each purification step and assess the degree of purity of the final product. As shown below, SE-HPLC is particularly well suited for these purposes. Since size exclusion separations are based on molecular weight, results are highly reproducible and not subject to variations due to charge differences among different monoclonal antibodies or even among different batches of the same antibody. Because of the high detection sensitivity of HPLC systems, acceptable chromatograms can be obtained with a minimum of sample and in a short time.

1. Determination of IgG Monoclonal Antibodies Concentration in Mouse Ascites

A preliminary indication of the feasibility of using SE-HPLC for this purpose is given by the separation of the Bio-Rad gel filtration protein standard mixture in a Bio-Sil® TSK 250 column (Bio-Rad Laboratories, Richmond, CA. 94804) (Fig. 1, Panel A). A good separation is obtained between bovine IgG, 158,000 MW (peak 2) and ovalbumin, 44,000 MW (peak 3). Since albumin is usually the main contaminant in mouse ascites, the data suggested that a satisfactory separation between albumin and monoclonal antibody IgG could also be obtained with mouse ascites samples. Figure 1, panel B, shows that this is the case. When SE-HPLC was performed with mouse ascites containing IgG_1 monoclonal antibody, two well-defined peaks (peaks 2 and 3) are observed at the positions of IgG and albumin, respectively. As shown before (2), mouse ascites contains no other major proteins eluting at the peak 2 position. Thus, the area or height of this peak can be used to calculate the IgG concentration in mouse ascites samples. Figure 2 shows a standard curve generated by measuring the peak 2 height from SE-HPLC chromatograms obtained by injecting 10 μl of a sample containing 2, 4, 6, 8, and 10 mg/ml of a purified IgG standard. A linear relationship between peak height and IgG concentration is observed within this range. Once the standard curve is generated, the IgG concentration of mouse ascites samples can be easily calculated. Obviously this method is also useful for calculating IgG yields during and after purification or to monitor the efficiency of a given purification procedure, as shown in Section III.

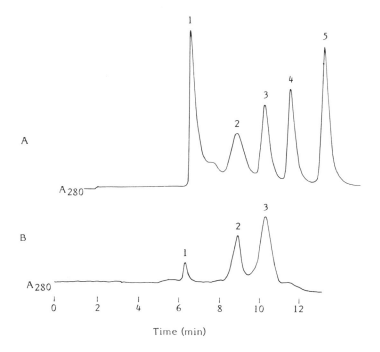

Figure 1 Panel A. SE-HPLC of Bio-Rad's gel filtration protein standard mixture containing: thyroglobulin, 670,000 MW (peak 1); bovine IgG, 158,000 MW (peak 2); chicken ovalbumin, 44,000 MW (peak 3); horse myoglobinim, 17,000 MW (peak 4), and vitamin B-12, 1,350 MW (peak 5). Panel B. SE-HPLC of mouse ascites containing an IgG monoclonal antibody. In both experiments, chromatography was performed using a Quick Check Analyzer HPLC system equipped with a Bio-Sil TSK 250 column set (300 × 7.5 mm analytical column; 75 × 7.5 mm guard column) and a 1306 variable wavelength UV monitor (Bio-Rad Laboratories, Richmond, CA 94804). Chromatography was performed isocratically, by injecting 10 μl of sample into the HPLC system. Absorbance was monitored at 280 nm. Flow rate was 1 ml/min. Chart speed was 60 cm/hr. Mobile phase was 10 mM sodium phosphate, 0.3 M NaCl pH 6.8 buffer containing 10% (v/v) dimethylsulfoxide.

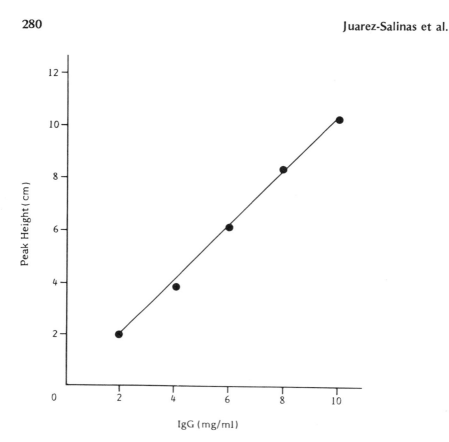

Figure 2 SE-HPLC IgG standard curve. Curve was generated by measuring the peak height of the IgG peak from SE-HPLC chromatograms obtained with increasing concentrations of Bio-Rad's purified bovine IgG standard. HPLC instrumentation and parameters were the same as indicated in Figure 1.

2. Determination of Monoclonal Antibody Class

Another characteristic of SE-HPLC is its ability to differentiate between samples containing IgG and IgM monoclonal antibody. Figure 3 shows the SE-HPLC profile of ascites containing either an IgG (panel A) or an IgM (panel B) monoclonal antibody. Two main differences in the profiles are readily apparent. First, the profile from the IgM-containing ascites (panel B) is devoid of peak 2, usually present in IgG-containing ascites (panel A). Second, panel B peak 1 is almost as large as the albumin peak. This peak is relatively small in IgG-containing ascites (panel A). Peak 1 represents the position of elution of high molecular weight proteins (above 500,000 MW)

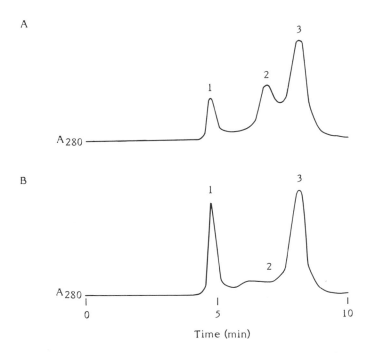

Figure 3   Panel A. SE-HPLC of mouse ascites containing an IgG monoclonal antibody. Panel B. SE-HPLC of mouse ascites containing an IgM monoclonal antibody. Chromatograms were obtained with 10 μl of mouse ascites as indicated in Figure 1, panel B.

such as IgM, which are totally excluded in the TSK 250 column. The presence of IgM in panel B peak 1 was confirmed using enzyme-linked immunosorbent assays (ELISA) for both IgM and antigen recognition (data not shown). The presence of other proteins besides IgM in peak 1 hinders the use of this procedure for quantitative determinations. Therefore this technique is recommended only for qualitative applications.

Although the SE-HPLC data presented here were obtained with mouse ascites fluid, the same methodology can be applied to tissue culture medium. However, in serum-supplemented tissue culture medium the concentration of albumin is usually many times larger than the concentration of the monoclonal antibody, making it difficult, if not impossible, to visualize the IgG peak. In these cases, a preliminary step, aimed at the reduction of the albumin concentration, such as ammonium sulfate precipitation or DEAE-blue agarose chromatography, is recommended. When serum-free tissue culture medium is used, control SE-HPLC profiles of the virgin medium should be obtained.

III. PURIFICATION OF MONOCLONAL ANTIBODIES

Frequently the purification of monoclonal antibodies is complicated by the fact that the starting material is contaminated with extraneous immunoglobulin molecules (3–5). These immunoglobulins may arise from the host mouse in the case of hybridomas grown in ascites fluid, from serum-supplemented tissue culture medium, or from the hybridoma itself, as in the case of multiple light or heavy chain producer hybridomas. Therefore the purification scheme should not only be able to produce a pure immunoglobulin preparation but also be able to separate the monoclonal antibody from the contaminating immunoglobulins. As shown below, the purification of the immunoglobulin fraction from monoclonal-antibody-containing samples can be rapidly achieved with PA-HPLC. Further purification, in terms of separation of the monoclonal antibody from contaminating immunoglobulins, is achieved by HPHT.

A. Protein A High Performance Liquid Chromatography (PA-HPLC)

It is generally accepted that affinity chromatography with protein A from *Staphylococcus aureus* yields the purest immunoglobulin preparations (6). Figure 4 shows the high degree of purification routinely achieved with protein A chromatography as shown by sodium dodecyl sulfate polyacrylamide gel electrophoresis (SDS-PAGE). Lane 1 shows the position of the SDS-PAGE protein standards. Lanes 2 and 3 shows the SDS-PAGE profile of an IgG_1-containing mouse ascites sample before and after protein A chromatography. Note that only the bands corresponding to the heavy and light immunoglobulin chains are observed in the protein A-purified sample. These results indicate that the protein A-purified immunoglobulin is highly pure. However, the application of protein A chromatography to the purification of monoclonal antibodies had been limited by its poor affinity for mouse IgG_1, IgM, and IgA immunoglobulins. These problems have been solved by the development of a new protein A binding buffer solution (Affi-Prep Protein A MAPS binding buffer), which promotes the binding of these immunoglobulins to Protein A. As shown in Table 1, capacities of up to 5–7 mg/ml of protein A packing material are achieved for IgG_1, IgM, and IgA monoclonal antibodies. These capacities are at least five times higher than those obtained using published protocols (7).

Another limitation of protein A column chromatography has been the lack of commercially available prepacked columns suitable for HPLC. This problem

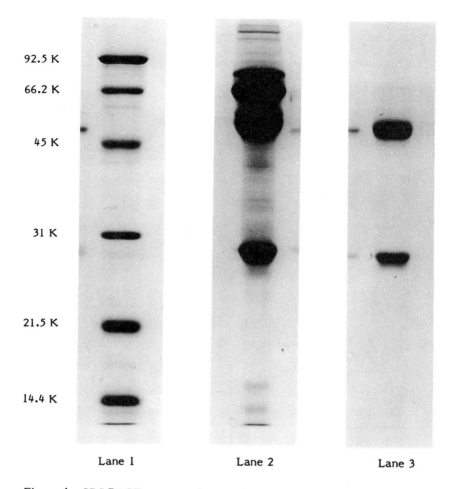

Figure 4   SDS-PAGE pattern of unpurified and protein A-purified IgG monoclonal antibody from mouse ascites. Lane 1, Bio-Rad SDS-PAGE molecular
weight standards; lane 2, unpurified mouse ascites; lane 3, protein A-purified
IgG monoclonal antibody. SDS-PAGE was performed by the method of
Laemmli (8). Proteins were stained with Coomassie blue.

Table 1 Affi-Prep[TM] Protein A HPLC
Columns and Cartridges[a]

Class	Capacity (mg mouse monoclonal antibody/ml matrix)
IgG$_1$	5.8
IgG$_{2A}$	8.3
IgG$_{2B}$	6.4
IgM	5.0
IgA	5.2

[a]The capacity of Affi-Prep protein A packing
material to bind IgG subclasses, IgM, and
IgA monoclonal antibodies is given in mg
antibody/ml packing material. This figure
should be used to calculate total column
capacity according to the column volume
figures given in Table 2. Affi-Prep protein
A is also available in bulk.

has been solved by the recent introduction of new polymer-based macro-
porous (1000 Å pore size) beads to which protein A has been chemically
cross-linked. (Affi-Prep protein A, Bio-Rad Laboratories, Richmond, CA
94804). Because of its high mechanical strength and porosity, this material
is ideal for use in the HPLC format. Table 2 lists the HPLC cartridges and
column sizes available. Cartridges with 0.5 and 7.5 ml volume capacity are
available for small and medium scale monoclonal antibody purification. Preparative chromatography with capacity to purify up to 250 mg IgG, IgM, or
IgA monoclonal antibodies can be performed with the 50 ml HPLC column.

1. IgG and IgM Monoclonal Antibody Purification

Affi-Prep protein A MAPS® typical chromatograms obtained with mouse
ascites containing either an IgG$_1$ or an IgM monoclonal antibody are shown
in Figure 5, panels A and B, respectively (MAPS Preparative System 100,
Bio-Rad Laboratories, Richmond, CA). Albumin and other impurities do not
bind to protein A and elute with the binding buffer wash (peak 1). Protein
A-bound immunoglobulins (peak 2) are eluted with elution buffer as indicated
by the arrow. Double peak patterns such as that observed in panel B, peak 2,
are usually caused by sample heterogeneity in terms of immunoglobulin composition. Notice that total chromatography time was only 15 min.

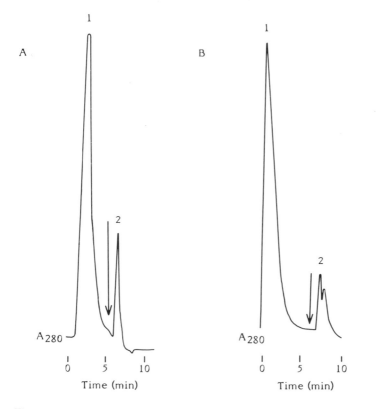

Figure 5   Panel A. Affi-Prep protein A MAPS chromatography of mouse ascites containing an IgG_1 monoclonal antibody. Panel B. Affi-Prep protein A MAPS chromatography of mouse ascites containing an IgM monoclonal antibody. In obth experiments 0.5 ml of mouse ascites containing 5 mg IgG_1 or 4 mg IgM monoclonal antibody was diluted 1:1 with Affi-Prep protein A MAPS binding buffer and injected into a MAPS preparative HPLC system equipped with a 4.6 X 100 mm Affi-Prep protein A column. Un-bound proteins were eluted with binding buffer (peak 1). Immunoglobulins were eluted with Affi-Prep protein A elution buffer at the time indicated by the arrow (peak 2). Flow rate was 0.5 ml/min. Absorbance was monitored at 280 nm.

Table 2   Affi-Prep Protein A HPLC
Column and Cartridges

	Dimensions (mm)	Volume (ml)
Cartridge	30 X 4.6	0.5
Cartridge	15 X 25	7.5
Column	100 X 25	50.0

The efficiency of the Affi-Prep protein A system to purify both mouse IgG_1 and mouse IgM monoclonal antibodies was explored by performing SE-HPLC of the protein A unbound and bound material (Figs. 6, 7). The SE-HPLC analysis of the protein A chromatography of the IgG_1-containing sample is shown in Figure 6. For comparison, the SE-HPLC profile from the mouse ascites prior to protein A chromatography is shown in panel A. Notice that the IgG peak (peak 2) is clearly visible. Chromatogram B shows the SE-HPLC profile of the protein A-unbound material. The IgG peak (peak 2) is almost completely absent, while peaks 1 and 3 are unaffected. This result indicates that the protein A cartridge has efficiently retained the IgG immunoglobulin present in the sample. The protein A-bound material was then eluted and analyzed by SE-HPLC (panel C). Only peak 2 is observed, indicating that the immunoglobulin isolated by protein A chromatography is highly pure.

Figure 7 shows the SE-HPLC chromatograms of the IgM-containing mouse ascites. Again, for comparison, panel A shows the SE-HPLC profile of mouse ascites prior to protein A chromatography. Notice that the IgG peak (peak 2) is absent while a large peak is observed at the IgM position (peak 1). Panel B shows the profile of the material not retained by the protein A cartridge. Notice the drastic reduction in the relative size of peak 1. Panel C shows the profile of the protein A retained fraction. Only one peak at the IgM position (peak 1) is observed. The identification of the protein A retained material as IgM was further corroborated by ELISA using polyclonal antimouse IgM immunoglobulin (data not shown).

These experiments show that IgG_1 and IgM monoclonal antibodies can be conveniently purified with PA-HPLC. Since other mouse IgG subclasses (IgG_{2A}, IgG_{2B}, and IgG_3) are known to bind to protein A with high efficiency, the Affi-Prep protein A MAPS system is essentially applicable to most of the existing monoclonal antibodies.

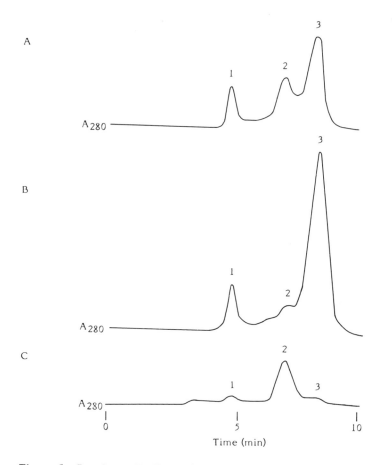

Figure 6 Panel A. SE-HPLC of mouse ascites containing an IgG$_1$ mono-clonal antibody before Affi-Prep protein A MAPS chromatography. Panel B. SE-HPLC of protein A-unbound material. Panel C. SE-HPLC of protein A-bound IgG. Conditions are described in Figure 1 legend.

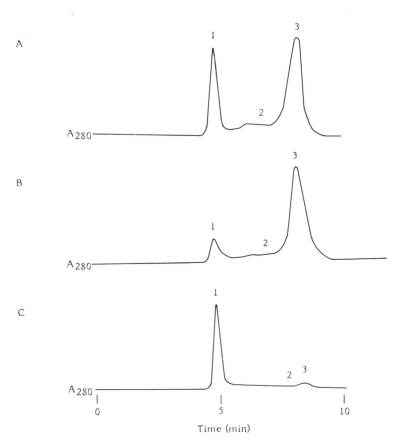

Figure 7 Panel A. SE-HPLC of mouse ascites containing an IgM monoclonal antibody before Affi-Prep protein A MAPS chromatography. Panel B. Protein A-unbound material. Panel C. Protein A-bound IgM. Conditions are described in Figure 1 legend.

B. High-Performance Hydroxylapatite Chromatography (HPHT)

Once the immunoglobulin fraction containing the monoclonal antibody has been satisfactorily purified by PA-HPLC, it is frequently necessary to separate the active monoclonal antibody from the inactive immunoglobulins. This section shows two examples of the use of HPHT chromatography (Bio-Rad Laboratories, Richmond, CA) to perform this separation. Example 1 deals with the separation of the active monoclonal antibody from other inactive or partially active immunoglobulin produced by the same hybridoma. Example 2 shows the ability of HPHT chromatography to separate a human monoclonal antibody from the bovine immunoglobulin present in fetal calf serum-supplemented tissue culture medium. The experiments presented here were performed with an analytical HPHT column (100 × 7.8 mm). Larger columns with up to 250 mg capacity for immunoglobulin are available for preparative work, as shown in Table 3 (Bio-Rad Laboratories, Richmond, CA).

1. Separation of Monoclonal Antibody Light Chain Variants

Figure 8 shows the HPHT profiles of protein A-purified H-1 monoclonal antibody. This antibody is directed against a human hemoglobin epitope and belongs to the IgG_{2A}, lambda light chain subclass. The chromatogram shows the presence of three peaks. Each one of these peaks was shown to contain immunoglobulins of the IgG_{2A} lambda light chain by ELISA. When the ability of peaks 1, 2, and 3 to recognize hemoglobin was tested, it was found that peak 1 was inactive, peak 2 was mildly active, and peak 3 was fully active (Fig. 9). These results suggest that the hybridoma that produced the H-1 antibody might be synthesizing different immunoglobulin molecules. To investigate this possibility, the protein A-purified MAb was subjected to reducing SDS-PAGE before and after HPHT chromatography. Figure 10 shows the SDS-PAGE pattern obtained with purified H-1 immunoglobulin. While only one band was observed in the heavy band region, two light chain

Table 3   HPHT MAPS: Columns and Cartridges

	Dimensions (mm)	Volume (ml)	Capacity IgG, IgM (mg/ml matrix)
Cartridge	30 × 4.6	0.5	5.0
Column	100 × 7.8	5.0	50.0
Column	50 × 25	25.0	250.0

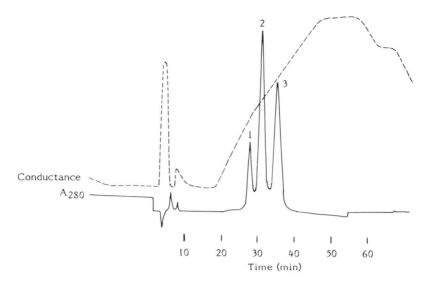

Figure 8 HPHT chromatography of protein A-purified H-1 monoclonal anti-body. Protein A-purified IgG was dialyzed against 10 mM sodium phosphate, pH 6.8 buffer (buffer A). Two milliliters of dialysate containing 2 mg pure H-1 IgG was filtered through a 0.22 μm membrane filter prior to chromato-graphy. HPHT was performed in a MAPS preparative HPLC system equipped with a Bio-Gel column set (7.8 X 100 mm analytical column and a 7.8 X 30 mm guard column; Bio-Rad Laboratories, Richmond, CA 94804). After sample application, the column was washed with 20 ml buffer A. IgG was eluted with a 30 min gradient from 10 mM sodium phosphate, pH 6.8 to 300 mM sodium phosphate, pH 6.8 (buffer B). Flow rate was 1 ml/min. (___) Absorbance at 280 nm; (---) conductivity.

bands were observed. These light chains were designated slow and fast migrating light chains. Figure 11, lanes 1, 2, and 3 (from left to right), shows the SDS-PAGE pattern of HPHT peaks 1, 2, and 3 from Figure 7. Lane 1 contained only the slow migrating light chain; lane 2 shows the presence of both the slow and the fast migrating light chain; peak 3 con-tained only the fast migrating light chain. Thus, these results support the theory that the multiple peaks separated by HPHT chromatography represent different immunoglobulin molecules produced by the intracellular presence of two different light chains. This situation is observed when light chain-producing myeloma cell lines are used in the original fusion in which the hybridoma was produced. A schematic representation of the putative immunoglobulin species produced by H-1 hybridoma is presented in Figure 12.

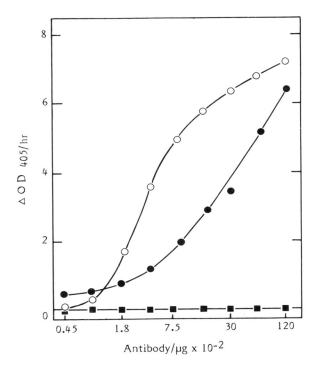

Figure 9   Antihuman hemoglobin activity of hydroxylapatite peaks 1, 2, and 3. A sample from each peak was assayed for antihemoglobin activity using ELISA. Peak 1 (square), peak 2 (circle), and peak 3 (open circle).

Immunoglobulins from peaks 1 and 3 are composed of two heavy chains and two either slow or fast migrating light chains, while peak 2 is a hybrid containing two heavy chains and one each of the slow and fast migrating light chains. These structures correlate well with the antibody activity determinations shown in Figure 8. The hybrid species shows intermediate activity, as is expected from a situation in which only one of the antibody arms recognizes the antigen, while peak 1 and 3 are either inactive or fully active depending on the presence of one or the other light chains.

2. Purification of Monoclonal Antibody from
    Polyclonal Fetal Calf Serum IgG

Hybridomas are frequently grown in tissue culture medium supplemented with fetal calf serum. Since fetal calf serum contains maternal IgG, purification of monoclonal antibodies from serum-supplemented tissue culture medium is

Heavy chain

Slow-migrating light chain

Fast-migrating light chain

Figure 10 SDS-PAGE of protein A-purified H-1 IgG. Pure H-1 immuno-globulin, 20 μg, was loaded into 10% gels. H-1 IgG was separated in three bands. One band (50,000 MW) corresponded to the IgG heavy chain. The other two bands (25,000 MW) corresponded to the slow- and fast-migrating light chains. Electrophoresis was performed by the method of Laemmli (8). Proteins were stained with Coomassie blue.

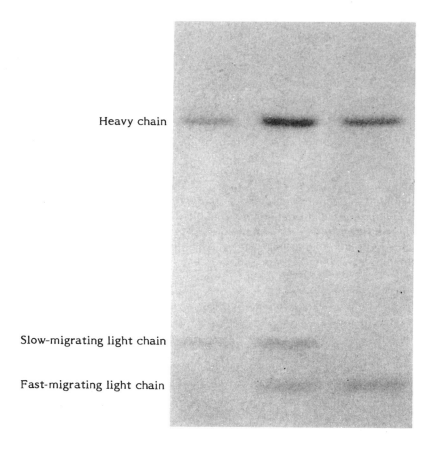

Figure 11 SDS-PAGE of HPHT peaks. Peaks 1, 2, and 3 from the experiment shown in Figure 8 were collected and concentrated by ultrafiltration. Approximately 10 μg from each peak was used for electrophoresis. Peak 1 contained only the slow-migrating light chain (lane 1, from left to right); peak 2 was a hybrid containing the slow- and the fast-migrating light chain (lane 2), and peak 3 contained only the fast-migrating light chain (lane 3).

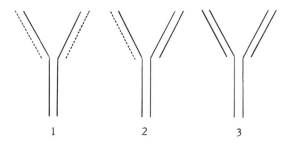

Figure 12 Schematic illustration of the proposed structures of H-1 immunoglobulins as separated by HPHT chromatography (Fig. 8). HPHT peak 1 contained only the myeloma-derived light chain; HPHT peak 2 contained is a
hybrid containing both the myeloma and the B-cell-derived light chain, while
HPHT peak 3 contained only the B-cell-derived light chain.

complicated by the presence of bovine polyclonal IgG. The following set of
results illustrate the ability of HPHT chromatography to separate a human
monoclonal antibody from fetal calf serum IgG. In order to have an appropriate control, bovine IgG was first isolated directly from fetal calf serum
using protein A chromatography. A second protein A chromatography was
then performed with monoclonal antibody-containing tissue culture medium
supplemented with 10% of the same fetal calf serum. Both samples were
then chromatographed on HPHT. Figure 13, panel A, shows the HPHT
profile obtained with purified fetal calf serum IgG. As expected, a broad
immunoglobulin peak representing the polyclonal IgG population is observed
instead of the sharp narrow peaks usually obtained with monoclonal antibodies. Figure 13, panel B, shows the HPHT profile obtained with serum-
supplemented tissue culture medium containing the monoclonal antibody.
Two peaks are observed, the first peak (peak 1) is similar to the panel A
profile and therefore represents the bovine IgG polyclonal population, while
the second narrower peak (peak 2) eluting late in the gradient presumably
represents the human monoclonal antibody. To establish the identity of
peak 2, fractions were collected and scanned for the presence of human
immunoglobulin and antigen recognition ability by ELISA, as shown in
Figure 14. Both human immunoglobulin and antigen recognition activity
are concentrated in peak 2. The data demonstrate once more the ability of
HPHT chromatography to differentiate between different immunoglobulin
molecules.

A.

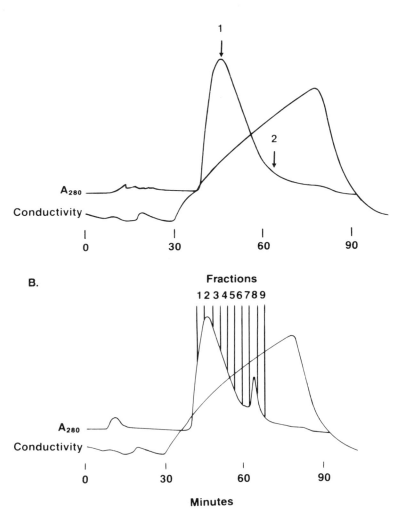

B.

Fractions
123456789

Minutes

Figure 13 Separation of a human IgG$_1$ monoclonal antibody from fetal calf serum IgG. Panel A. HPHT profile of protein A-purified fetal calf serum IgG. Panel B. HPHT profile from protein-A purified fetal calf serum supplemented (10%) tissue culture medium containing the human monoclonal antibody. Nine fractions were collected as indicated. HPHT chromatography was performed as indicated in Figure 8.

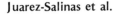
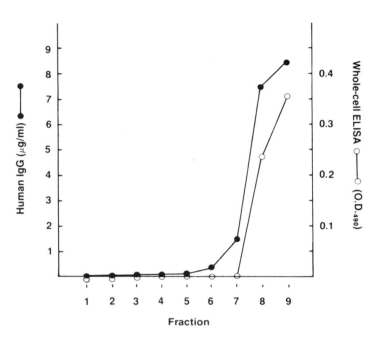

Figure 14 Determination of human IgG and antigen recognition in Figure 13, panel B fractions. The ability to recognize a cell surface antigen and the presence of human IgG were determined by ELISA in each of the fractions corresponding to peaks 1 and 2 from Figure 13, panel B.

IV. CONCLUSIONS

Monoclonal antibodies can be conveniently characterized and purified by HPLC. The monoclonal antibody class and concentration is first determined by size exclusion HPLC. This method is also used to monitor the efficiency of the purification process. Both IgG (including mouse IgG_1) and IgM monoclonal antibodies are first purified with protein A HPLC. This procedure yields a highly pure immunoglobulin preparation that contains the monoclonal antibody. A second chromatographic step with high performance hydroxylapatite separates the monoclonal antibody from contaminating immunoglobulin molecules. The HPLC sample preparations procedures for mouse ascites and tissue culture medium are presented in Appendix 5.

ACKNOWLEDGMENTS

This work was performed under the auspices of the Chromatography Business Unit, Chemical Division, Bio-Rad Laboratories. We wish to thank Mr. Christopher J. Siebert and Mr. Christopher Rew for helpful discussions during the course of this work.

REFERENCES

1. Kohler, G. and Milstein, C. (1975). Continuous cultures of fused cells secreting antibody of predefined specificity. *Nature 256*: 495–497.
2. Juarez-Salinas, H., Bigbee, W. L., LaMotte, G. B. III, and Ott, G. S. (1986, March/April). New procedures for the analysis and purification of IgG murine MAbs. *Am. Biotech. Lab.*
3. Juarez-Salinas, H., Ott, G. S., Chen, J.-C., Brooks, T. L., and Stanker, L. H. (1986). Separation of IgG idiotypes by high-performance hydroxylapatite chromatography. *Meth. Enzymol. 121*: 615.
4. Juarez-Salinas, H. Engelhorn, S. C., Bigbee, W. L., Lowry, M. A., and Stanker, L. H. (1984). Ultrapurification of monoclonal antibodies by high-performance hydroxylapatite (HPHT) chromatography. *BioTechniques 2*: 164–168.
5. Stanker, L. H., Vanderlaan, M., and Juarez-Salinas, H. (1985). One-step purification of mouse monoclonal antibodies from ascites fluid by hydroxylapatite chromatography. *J. Immunol. Meth. 76*: 157–169.
6. Langone, J. J. (1982). Applications of immobilized protein A in immunochemical techniques. *J. Immunol. Meth. 55*: 277–296.
7. Ey, P. L., Prowse, S. J., and Jenkin, C. R. (1978). Isolation of pure IgG_1, IgG_{2a} and IgG_{2b} immunoglobulins from mouse serum using protein A-sepharose. *Immunochemistry 15*: 429.
8. Laemmli, V. (1970). Cleavage of structural proteins during the assembly of the head of bacteriophage T4. *Nature 227*: 680–685.

APPENDIXES

Appendix 1

Federal Regulations Pertaining to the Production of Monoclonal Antibodies for In Vitro and In Vivo Uses

SALLY S. SEAVER
Hygeia Sciences, Newton, Massachusetts

In 1983 Dr. Bruce Merchant proposed guidelines for the production of monoclonal antibodies called "Points to Consider for Monoclonal Antibody Production." Numerous comments have been made on these proposed guidelines. Although no revised or final guidelines were issued, producers have incorporated these points into their manufacturing procedures. Recently, a new set of guidelines that focuses on the production of monoclonal antibodies for injection has been drafted and is under review. When this latest version is approved, it will be available through the Division of Blood and Blood Products, Office of Biological Research and Review, Center for Drugs and Biologics (DBBP,OBRR,CDB), HFN-838, 8800 Rockville Pike, Bethesda, Maryland 20892. The current director is Dr. Thomas Hoffman (Phone: 301-496-4538). Dr. Hoffman is also the author of several articles on regulatory issues involved in the production of monoclonal antibodies (1,2).

In March 1986, Dr. Edward McDonnell, Director of the Division of Compliance Programs, Center for Devices and Radiological Health, HFZ-332, 8757 Georgia Avenue, Silver Springs, Maryland 20910, issued a working draft of "In Vitro Diagnostic Devices—Inspectional Guidelines" for comments. This document contains points that should be considered during culturing of any cell line or virus, including hybridoma cells.

In addition to these specific guidelines, the production of monoclonal antibodies for diagnostic, therapeutic, or manufacturing purposes must be done under good manufacturing practices and must involve clearance of the final product with the appropriate regulatory agencies.

REFERENCES

1. Hoffman, T., Kenimer, J., and Stein, K. E. (1985). Regulatory issues sur-rounding therapeutic uses of monoclonal antibodies. Points to consider in the manufacturing of injectible products intended for human use. In *Monoclonal Antibodies and Cancer Therapy*. UCLA Symposium on Molecular and Cellular Biology. Edited by R. A. Reisfeldt and S. Sell. New York, Alan R. Liss, pp. 431–440.
2. Hoffman, T. (1987). Regulatory issues surrounding therapeutic uses of monoclonal antibody. In *Hybridoma Formation*. Edited by A. Bartal and Y. Hirshault. Humana Press, Clifton, NJ, pp. 447–456.

Appendix 2
Procedure for Using Protein A-Sepharose CL-4B to Purify Monoclonal Antibody

SHWU-MAAN LEE*

Program Resources, Inc., National Cancer Institute–Frederick Cancer Research Facility, National Institutes of Health, Frederick, Maryland

Protein A-Sepharose CL-4B was used to purify a mouse IgG_{2a} monoclonal antibody from tissue culture supernatant. The column used here can produce 2–4 g antibody each cycle. The tight binding between IgG and protein A allows the removal of protein contaminant and endotoxins. However, this method does not work well with weakly bound antibodies.

I. MATERIALS

1. Pellicon ultrafiltration system (Millipore) with polysulfone membrane cassette (100,000 NMWCO[†]).
2. Sealkleen Zeta potential filters, 2 μm and 0.22 μm (Pall).
3. Protein A-Sepharose CL-4B (Pharmacia), hydrated in water or 0.05 M potassium phosphate buffer, pH 7.0, containing 0.2 M NaCl.
4. Sepharose CL-4B (Pharmacia).
5. All the solutions used for antibody purification and column regeneration were sterile filtered with Millistak GS 0.22 μm filters (Millipore).
6. K 100/45 column (Pharmacia) for protein A–Sepharose CL-4B.
7. BP 113/15 column (Pharmacia, 11.3 cm in diameter with adjustable bed height) for Sepharose CL-4B; this is the recommended size for a precolumn.

Present affiliation: Genex Corporation, Gaithersburg, Maryland.
†Nominal molecular weight cut-off.

8. The glassware was cleaned with 1% nitric acid after detergent washing and autoclaved.

II. PROCEDURE

1. Concentrate antibody from cell culture supernatant (280 L/run) 10–20-fold using the Pellicon ultrafiltration system with 25 ft.^{2} polysulfone membrane. Specific details of Pellicon operation have been described by William B. Lebherz III in Chapter 6.
2. Clarify antibody concentrate with 2 μm Sealkleen Zeta potential filters and store as frozen aliquots.
3. Set up protein A-Sepharose CL-4B column (10 cm × 7 cm) and Sepharose CL-4B precolumn (11.3 cm × 3 cm) at 2–8°C. A linear flow rate of 52 cm/hr was maintained at an operating pressure of 0.25 bar. Store the column in 0.02% sodium azide.
4. Wash the column with depyrogenated water until less than 0.1 ppm azide is detected in the effluent (1).
5. Equilibrate the column with 0.05 M potassium phosphate buffer containing 0.2 M NaCl, pH 8.4 (PBS).
6. Thaw antibody concentrate at 2–8°C, adjusted to pH 8.4 with 2 M KOH and adsorb onto the column.
7. Wash the column with PBS, pH 8.4 (10–15 L), and elute with 0.05 M monobasic potassium phosphate containing 0.2 M NaCl, pH 4.5.
8. Regenerate the column with 3 M KSCN after each use. After a few cycles, further clean the column with 0.05 M potassium phosphate, pH 8.5, containing 0.5 M NaCl, and 0.05 M monobasic potassium phosphate, pH 4.5, containing 0.5 M NaCl.
9. Adjust the eluent fractions to pH 7.0–7.4 with 2 M KOH and store them at −30°C.
10. Thaw the antibody-rich column fractions at 2–8°C and pool them. Concentrate the pool to the desired protein concentration using the Pellicon ultrafiltration system.
11. Determine the chloride concentration and adjust to 0.5 M with NaCl.
12. Filter the formulated antibody solution through a 0.2 μm Sealkleen filter into sterile glass bottles.
13. Store the bulk, sterile product at 2–8°C.

REFERENCE

1. *United States Pharmacopeia.* 21st revision (1985). United States Pharmacopeial Convention, Inc., p. 1187.

Appendix 3

Procedures for Using ABx to Purify Antibody

DAVID R. NAU
J. T. Baker Chemical Company, Phillipsburg, New Jersey

This Appendix describes the procedures for using and maintaining the BAKER-BOND ABx bulk bonded phases and HPLC columns. ABx is available from J. T. Baker Chemical Company (Phillipsburg, New Jersey) in the following configurations: prepacked HPLC columns containing 5 μm ABx or MAb in the "analytical" (4.6 × 250 mm), "GOLD" (7.75 × 100 mm [FPLC compatible]), "prep" (10 × 250 mm) or custom (any size) column configurations; prepacked HPLC (FPLC-compatible) columns containing 15 μm ABx or MAb in the "prep" (10 × 250 mm) or custom (any size) column configuration; 5 and 15 μm ABx or MAb bulk bonded phases for "topping off" old HPLC columns or for slurry (pressure) packing into HPLC columns; 40 μm ABx and MAb bulk bonded phases for batch extractions and for traditional open column (low pressure) chromatography; and ABx and MAb spe™ columns for rapid sample preparation/clean-up.

I. HYGIENE: CLEAN–UP, REGENERATION, AND STERILIZATION

If column performance deteriorates unexpectedly, or if column back-pressure increases substantially, column clean-up may be required to remove adsorbed proteins or lipids. ABx and MAb may be regenerated with 20 column volumes of high-ionic-strength salt solutions, such as 2M sodium acetate or 1M potassium phosphate buffer, pH 7 or 8, using high flow rates. If necessary, further washes may be carried out with 10 column volumes of protein solubilizing agents such as 5M urea or guanidine; detergents such as 1%

305

Triton X-100, SDS, or Brij 35; acids such as 0.2% trifluoroacetic acid, 1% acetic acid, or 1% formic acid; or organic solvents such as methanol, or 50:50 DMSO:H_2O (to remove lipids).

At the end of each day it is advisable to store the column in a high salt buffer to clean off contaminants and prevent microbial growth. Unlike most polysaccharide-based soft gels, silica-based bonded phases themselves do not support the growth of microorganisms, although microbial growth may occur in low-ionic-strength mobile phases. Therefore, if the column is to be stored for long periods (more than a week), the use of pure methanol, ethanol, propanol or a preservative such as 0.1% sodium azide or chlorhexidine in high-ionic-strength buffer (1M KH_2PO_4, 2M $(NH_4)_2SO_4$, or 2M NaOAc, pH 7.0) is recommended. The column may also be refrigerated. Columns are typically stable for over 1,000 hr of use at room temperature. Dry ABx and MAb bulk bonded phases need not be refrigerated and are extremely stable.

Sterilization of ABx and MAb columns or bulk bonded phases may be accomplished by washing with any bactericidal organic solvent such as ethanol, methanol, acetonitrile, or a 0.1% aqueous solution of sodium azide or chlorhexidine. The ABx and MAb matrices are unaffected by and totally resistant to these treatments.

Although ABx and MAb media are silica-based, their dense hydrophilic polymeric coverage allows for the use of pH extremes (2–10) not permitted with most other silica-based materials. ABx and MAb are totally resistant to most organic solvents, aqueous buffers, chaotropic and protein solubilizing agents, detergents, antimicrobials, and bactericides.

II. COLUMN LIFETIME

Columns of ABx media have been use-tested for more than 1,000 hr without appreciable loss in resolution or capacity. Column lifetime may be optimized by using HPLC grade solvents and salts. Solvent filtering (with 0.5 μm filters) and the use of inline filters or guard columns is also desirable. Biological samples should be passed through 0.5 μm filters or at least centrifuged prior to injection to remove microorganisms and other debris and to avoid clogging column frits. Prolonged exposure to extremes in pH should also be avoided although pHs between 2 and 10 may be successfully used for extended periods. Column regeneration procedures should also be followed if changes in resolution, capacity, or retention times occur (see above).

III. BATCH EXTRACTION WITH ABx

The protocol for the batch extraction of cell culture supernatant with 40 μm PREPSCALE ABx (Fig. 1) is as follows. About 40 mg 40 μm PREPSCALE

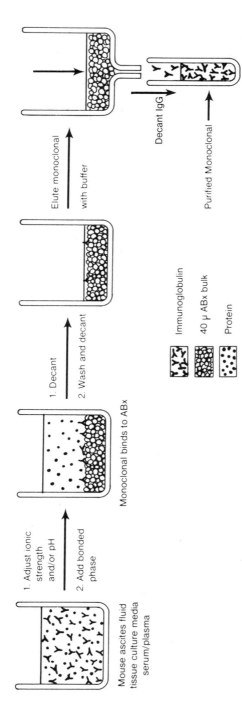

Figure 1 Batch extraction schematic—BAKERBOND ABx.

ABx bonded phase is slurried in 10 mM MES buffer, pH 5.6. After being stirred for several minutes or sonicated (optional) for 30 sec, the buffer is removed by decanting or filtration. A 5 ml sample of diluted cell culture supernatant (1 ml supernatant ultrafiltrate diluted with 4 ml 10 mM MES, pH 5.60) is added to the bonded phase. After the slurry is gently stirred for 5 min the supernatant is removed (ABx settles rapidly by gravity). The remaining bonded phase is first washed with 2 ml 10 mM MES, pH 5.6, and then extracted with 2 ml 200 mM KH_2PO_4, pH 7.4. At least 70% of the immunoglobulin present in the original sample is now present in this buffer. Supernatants at each step of the extraction procedure may be analyzed for immunoglobulin using a column packed with 5 μm ABx, or by traditional means of antibody analysis (SDS PAGE, gel filtration, protein A, ELISA, etc.). The method can be optimized further by using a larger quantity of bonded phase, higher molarities to desorb the IgG, and/or by recycling the unadsorbed immunoglobulin from the first extraction in further extraction cycles.

IV. SOLID PHASE EXTRACTION WITH ABx

Solid phase extraction (spe) is a rapid method for sample preparation and/or sample clean-up using small polyethylene columns containing 0.5 g packing material. Unlike conventional column chromatography, with spe, the compound of interest (e.g., an antibody) is bound rather selectively, while the contaminants do not bind, and elute during the sample loadings. The compound of interest may then be desorbed into a small volume of buffer in a substantially purified state.

BAKERBOND ABx spe columns operate in a manner similar to affinity matrices by rather selectively removing immunoglobulins from crude biological mixtures. This procedure is useful for IgG enrichment, for ascites fluid screening, and for the fractionation of antibodies from animal serum. Note that this particular method is not designed to give high yield or purity, but rather to act as a quick sample clean-up method.

The ABx spe column is conditioned by aspirating with 15 ml buffer A (10 mM phosphate buffer, pH 5.5). The sample is prepared by diluting one part of ascites fluid (0.5 ml) with nine parts of buffer A. This is aspirated through the column, which is then washed with 5 ml buffer A. The IgG is eluted with 2 ml buffer B (200 mM phosphate buffer, pH 7.5). Typically, the IgG recovery is 65% and the IgG enrichment is 70% as determined by HPLC (Fig. 2) and SDS PAGE. This procedure was developed using mouse ascites and human plasma and serum. For samples from other animal sources the molarities of buffers A and B may differ slightly for optimal results. Buffers other than phosphate (Sections VII and VIII) may also be used with molarity adjustments to maintain appropriate ionic strengths.

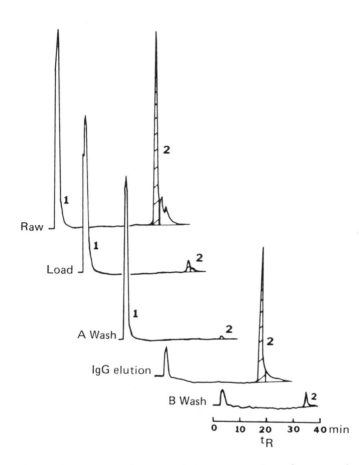

Figure 2 Results of the solid-phase extraction of a monoclonal antibody from mouse ascites fluid using BAKERBOND ABx spe columns as analyzed by ABx HPLC column chromatography. Analytical conditions are given in Figure 3 of Chapter 13. Peak 1, albumin and transferrin; peak 2, IgG.

V. SAMPLE PREPARATION

Ionic strength must be relatively low to maximize the binding of antibodies to ABx. Any technique may be used for this, including dialysis, membrane ultrafiltration or dilution. The optimal sample pH may vary with individual samples, but dilution of the sample with or ultrafiltration or dialysis against a zwitterionic buffer of low ionic strength at pH 5.0-6.0 (e.g., 10-25 mM MES

(2-[N-morpholino]-ethane sulfonic acid) or MOPSO (3-[N-morpholino]-2-hydroxypropane sulfonic acid), pH 5.6) is generally suitable.

VI. ABx CAPACITY AND SAMPLE LOADING

The binding capacity of 5 μm ABx is approximately 150 mg purified IgG/g bonded phase (breakthrough method), corresponding to a titration of about 0.4 mEq/g packing. The ligand titrations of the 15 and 40 μm (PREPSCALE) preparative media are higher (approximately 0.7 mEq/g and 1.0 mEq/g, respectively), due to their higher surface areas and lower densities (Table 2, Chapter 13).

Loading capacities on ABx columns, of course, depend upon the nature of the sample. Higher ionic strength, pH, total protein contents, and levels of immunoglobulin and other "bound" proteins all reduce the amount of sample that can be loaded onto the column for quantitative binding of the antibody. Therefore, dialysis, dilution, or, particularly, ultrafiltration against the ABx starting (A) buffer is recommended to reduce the amount of antibody not bound to the column due to displacement chromatography by proteins, and salts present within the sample itself. Tangential flow ultrafiltration is valuable due to its ability to concentrate large volumes of culture medium into starting (A) buffer, and to reduce the concentration of nonimmunoglobulin proteins in the process, decreasing the total amount of protein more than 10-fold in many cases.

For example, sample loads as high as 30 ml serum-based tissue culture medium (6 ml 20-fold concentrated ultrafiltrate diluted fourfold with 10 mM MES pH 5.6) have been chromatographed on ABx columns (4.6 $\times$ 250 mm) containing 1.0 g packing (Fig. 1, Chapter 13), with greater than 80% of the IgG binding (75 ml of the same sample produced a 70% recovery of the IgG). Obviously, the unbound void volume fraction containing the displaced IgG (20%) can be directly recycled onto the same column in a second run to give greater than 96% recovery of the original IgG (20% of 20% is only 4% "lost").

Another example of sample loading is shown in Figure 2, Chapter 13, with 1.5 L of the same culture medium concentrate as above, which was chromatographed on a column containing 15 g 40 μm (PREPSCALE) ABx. In this case, more than 90% of the total IgG bound to the column, indicating that antibody binding is a function of column dimension as well as the amount of packing used for a given separation.

VII. STARTING BUFFERS

Columns are equilibrated with approximately 15 column volumes of starting buffer (10–25 mM MES, pH 5.6). This may be accomplished more quickly by beginning the equilibration with 50 mM MES, pH 5.6, and then switching to lower ionic strength MES (10 mM, pH 4.6).

MES (or MOPSO) buffer is typically used as the starting buffer, since zwitterionic buffers facilitate the binding of antibodies to the zwitterionic surface of ABx. Furthermore, pH equilibration may be conveniently monitored by following absorbance at 220 nm due to the change in absorbtivity (extinction coefficient) of MES that accompanies column pH equilibration. Alternatively, the pH of the column effluent may be monitored to determine when the column is equilibrated.

VIII. ELUTION BUFFERS

As indicated in Chapter 13, Section VIII, the use of various final (B) buffers results in different elution profiles from ABx (Fig. 5, Chapter 13). Four basic elution buffers (Table 1), each at pH 5.6 or 7.0, are recommended, although a variety of buffer species concentrations and pH values may be used successfully. For initial method development, it is suggested that 500 mM NaOAc, pH 7.0, be used, since the antibody elutes as a sharp peak in a low volume of eluent and this facilitates SDS PAGE analysis and identification. This "fraction" may then be used as a standard to identify the antibody peak in the presence of other buffer systems.

Since the antibody peak is not as sharp when eluted with $(NH_4)_2SO_4$ buffer, initial method development is usually not conducted with this mobile phase, unless there is an antibody standard, or a very sensitive method of identification is available (i.e., an immunologic assay, or SDS PAGE with silver stain), or if the antibody level is high (i.e., greater than 300 $\mu g/ml$).

In addition to changing the elution buffer conditions, dramatic changes in elution profile and selectivity can be achieved on ABx by changing the starting (A) buffer species and pH, following sample loading and antibody binding. Therefore, the pH or ionic strength of the MES or MOPSO buffers may be changed (i.e., 20–50 mM MES or MOPSO at pH 5.0–8.0), or the initial buffer species may be changed to KH_2PO_4 or Tris, etc. (10–50 mM at pH 5.0–8.0).

IX. FLOW RATES FOR ABx COLUMN CHROMATOGRAPHY

Flow rates for sample introduction (loading) should be 50–70% of those used for actual chromatography to facilitate antibody binding. Flow rates during chromatography will vary depending upon the internal diameter (id) of the column (4.6 mm id use 0.3–1.0 ml/min, 7.75 mm id use 0.5–1.5 ml/min,

Table 1   Suggested ABx Gradients[a]

Buffer A	Buffer B
10 mM MES pH 5.6 (MES acid adjusted to pH 5.6 with NaOH)[b]	500 mM $(NH_4)_2SO_4$ plus 10 mM NaOAc, pH 5.6 or 7.0
10 mM MOPSO pH 5.6 (MOPSO acid adjusted to pH 5.6 with NaOH)[b]	500 mM NaOAc, pH 5.6 or 7.0
	500 mM KH_2PO_4, pH 5.6 or 7.0
	500 mM NaCl plus 10 mM NaOAc, pH 5.6 or 7.0

[a]Gradients may be linear from 1 to 3 hr (with IgGs eluting from 18 to 90 min), or with step gradients to enhance IgG resolution and reduce run times. Alternatively, the ionic strengths of buffer B may be reduced. The optimal chromatographic conditions may vary, but for initial experiments use those given in Figure 6, Chapter 13, and Appendix Section X.
[b]Other low ionic strength (10–25 mM) MES or MOPSO buffers (pH 5.0–6.0) may also be used.

10 mm use 2–5 ml/min, 20 mm use 7–20 ml/min, 40 mm use 30–100 ml/min, etc.). The lower flow rates are typically used to improve resolution (Section X).

X. OPTIMIZATION OF PURIFICATION

As indicated in the various chromatograms and in Sections III and IV of Chapter 13, each antibody preparation represents a unique purification problem. Furthermore, not every monoclonal or polyclonal is destined for the same use, and as such, purity requirements differ substantially.

Although many immunoglobulins elute from ABx as electrophoretically pure peaks, the optimization of purification may involve the "fine tuning" of several parameters. These include choosing the correct buffer conditions (Section VIII), using step gradients to reduce run time (Fig. 8, Chapter 13), reduced flow rates (Fig. 5, Chapter 13 and Section I), reduced gradient steepness or elution buffer concentration (Section VIII), and isocratic elution (Fig. 9, Chapter 13) in order to improve resolution.

In cases where extreme product purity is required or large sample volumes are being processed, a purification scheme comprised of several steps on ABx may be required. Initial chromatography may be conducted on a larger column containing 40 μm PREPSCALE ABx using traditional, open-column chromatographic equipment. Since greater than 95% of the nonimmunoglobulin proteins will be removed in this first step, the second step is typically conducted on a much smaller HPLC column containing high-resolution 5 μm ABx and in the presence of a second buffer system (e.g., Fig. 5, Chapter 13). The active fractions may also be run isocratically in NaOAc buffer, pH 7.0, in order to maximize resolution (Fig. 9, Chapter 13). Again, use of the conditions detailed within the previous paragraph is suggested to optimize the separation.

Extremely high antibody purity may also be achieved with a combination of ABx and either a high-performance anion exchanger such as the MAb (Section X) or with a high-performance hydrophobic interaction chromatographic media such as BAKERBOND HI-Propyl. The latter is particularly suitable for the chromatographic separation of various immunoglobulin species and as a direct purification step following salt fractionation or ABx chromatography, since the antibody is bound in the presence of high salt concentrations, and as such, no sample dialysis/dilution is required.

In other cases, where product recovery is not a vital issue, batch extraction (for large sample volumes) or spe (for small sample volumes and/or numerous samples) may be adequate as an initial purification/clean-up step (Sections III and IV). Again, final step purification may be conducted on an ABx HPLC column.

Appendix 4
Rapid High-Performance Liquid Chromatography Technique for Monitoring Amino Acids in Culture Fluid

SALLY S. SEAVER
Hygeia Sciences, Newton, Massachusetts

Orthophthalaldehyde (OPA), in the presence of a mercaptan, reacts with primary amino acids to form fluorescent adducts. All primary amino acids, except cysteine, but not secondary amino acids proline and hydroxyproline, form stable derivatives which can be resolved by chromatography on C18 resin. The separation takes 30 min, requires no prior treatment of culture fluid, and can be automated. A more detailed description of this technique has been published previously (1).

I. MATERIALS

1. Fluoraldehyde (Pierce Chemicals) is a mixture of OPA, mercaptoethanol, and Brij-35 in a borate buffer. It is stored in the refrigerator. A drop of mercaptoethanol should be added every few days. If not, the positions of the peaks will be variable.
2. Organic free (amino acid free) water for buffers and diluting sample. Most distilled or deionized water has high levels of primary amines or glycine which react with OPA.

3. Buffer A: 0.05M sodium acetate, 0.05M sodium phosphate pH 7.4/ methanol/tetrahydrofuran, 96/2/2.
4. Buffer B: methanol/water, 65/35.
5. A Guard® column packed with C18 resin. This column, which is in front of the resolving column, binds the protein in the sample and extends the life of the resolving column. It should be changed every 50–100 injections.
6. Resolve® 5 μm C18 column (Waters Associates).
7. Amino Acid Standard Solution, AA-S-18, (Sigma Chemical Co.) contains all common primary amino acids except tryptophan, glutamine, and asparagine, which can be purchased separately from Sigma.
8. For manual operation one needs a sample injector, two pumps, a linear gradient maker, a fluorescent detector, a chart recorder, or data handling system such as Waters Associates' U-6K sample injector, M6000A solvent delivery systems, M721 System Controller, M420AC fluorescence detector, and M730 data module.
9. The above system can be automated with the addition of Water's Model 710 WISP® Sample Processor.

II. PROCEDURE

1. If desired, store the tissue culture medium at −20°C.
2. Equilibrate the Guard® C18 and Resolve® columns with Buffer A.
3. Dilute the culture fluid in organic-free water. A 50-fold dilution worked well with Dulbecco's Modified Eagle Medium/10% fetal bovine serum.
4a. For manual operation mix 100 μl diluted culture fluid with 200 μl fluoraldehyde. Let it react for 2 min before being injected onto the column.
4b. For automatic operation 10 μl diluted culture fluid is reacted with 20 μl fluoraldehyde (see program that follows.) The Guard® column with C18 resin should be as close to the WISP® as possible and should replace the "mixing" column.
5. The amino acid profile is generated by a 25 min linear gradient of 0–100% buffer B in buffer A at a flow rate of 1.5 ml/min.
6. The amino acid derivatives are detected with a 334 nm excitation filter and a 425 nm emission filter in the fluorometer.
7. The amino acids are quantified by measuring the area (not peak height) under each peak. Standard curves of peak heights versus amino acid concentration for specific amino acids are usually linear over the useful physiological range.

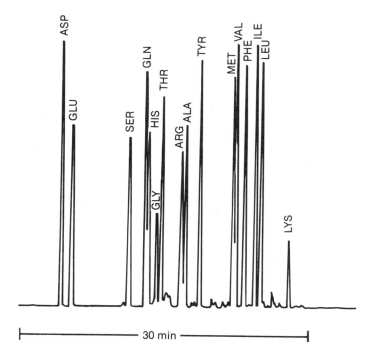

Figure 1   HPLC profile of the OPA derivatives of 16 of the primary amino acids commonly found in culture medium. ASP, aspartate; GLU, glutamate; SER, serine; GLN, glutamine; HIS, histidine; GLY, glycine; THR, threonine; ARG, arginine; ALA, alanine; TYR, tyrosine; MET, methionine; VAL, valine; PHE, phenylalanine; ILE, isoleucine; LYS, lysine. This profile does not contain tryptophan, which chromatographs between valine and phenylalanine or asparagine, which is just before serine. Secondary amino acids, proline and hydroxyproline, as well as cysteine do not form OPA derivatives.

Program for Automated Amino Acid Analysis

Step	Time (min)	Flow (ml/min)	Event
1	0	0	Inject 20 µl OPA, 10 µl sample, let them react for 2 min
2	2	<1.5	Linear ramp of pump speed to 1.5 ml/min with buffer A
3	3	1.5	Linear gradient to 100% buffer B (ends at 32 min)
4	32	1.5	8 min linear gradient to 100% buffer A
5	40	1.5	12 min wash of column with 100% buffer A
6	52	<1.5	Linear ramp of flow to 0 ml/min
7	53	0	Let column sit with no flow for 1 min

Step 7 is required to ensure that there is no residual pressure/flow of solvent during the injection/reaction step. If step 7 is omitted, the peak heights will be decreased because the residual pressure will force the OPA down the column before it is fully reacted with the sample.

REFERENCES

1. Seaver, S. S., Rudolph, J. L., and Gabriels, J. E. Jr. (1985). A rapid HPLC technique for monitoring amino acid utilization in cell culture. *BioTechniques 2*: 254–260.
2. Hill, D., Burnworth, L., Skea, W., and Pfeifer, R. (1982). Quantitative HPLC analysis of plasma amino acids as orthophthaldialdehyde/ethanethiol derivatives. *J. Liquid Chromatogr. 5*: 2369–2393.
3. Pfeifer, R. and Hill, D. W. (1983). High-performance liquid chromatography of amino acids: Ion-exchange and reversed-phase strategies. In *Advances in Chromatography*. Edited by J. C. Giddings, E. Grushka, J. Cazes, and P. R. Brown. New York, Marcel Dekker, *22*: 37–69.

Appendix 5

Sample Preparation Procedures for Mouse Ascitic Fluid and Tissue Culture Medium Before High-Performance Liquid Chromatography

HECTOR JUAREZ–SALINAS and TIMOTHY L. BROOKS
Bio-Rad Laboratories, Richmond, California

I. MOUSE ASCITIC FLUID

The following procedure is recommended for mouse ascites fluid before it is loaded into the HPLC systems.

1. After collection of the ascitic, promote conversion of fibrinogen to fibrin by adding enough concentrated $CaCl_2$ (100 mM) to reach a final concentration of 1 mM. This will accelerate the clotting process and allow clot removal before chromatography. The use of heparin to prevent clot formation is not recommended since heparin can be inadvertantly removed during the sample preparation procedure or during the chromatography process. The removal of heparin may result in clot formation inside the column.
2. Allow clot formation by keeping the ascites at room temperature for 2 hr.
3. Detach and remove the fibrin clot from the tube wall with a wooden applicator stick.
4. Store the ascites fluid overnight at 4°C.
5. Remove any new clots.
6. Remove cell debris by centrifugation at 10,000 X g for 30 minutes at 4°C.

7. Remove any remaining particulate material by centrifugation at 100,000 X g for 60 min at 4°C.*
8. Remove the lipid layer from the top of the sample.
9. Dilute or dialyze ascites appropriately depending upon the column chemistry to be used. For protein A-HPLC chromatography the sample is diluted 1:1 with Affi-Prep^{TM} protein A MAPS binding buffer.
10. Filter diluted ascites through a 0.22 μm filter just prior to injection into HPLC.

II. TISSUE CULTURE MEDIUM

Since the concentration of monoclonal antibodies in tissue culture medium is usually very low (10–100 μg/ml), it is convenient to subject the sample to a concentration step prior to chromatography. The following batch procedure based on the high capacity of hydroxylapatite powder (HTP, Bio-Rad Laboratories) to adsorb proteins is recommended.

1. Use 2.5 g hydroxylapatite for each 100 ml 10% serum-supplemented tissue culture medium or 1.25 g for each 100 ml serum-free tissue culture medium. Add the powder while the medium is being shaken or stirred.
2. Incubate 60 min with constant shaking or stirring.
3. Pour the suspension into a column. Wide columns (2.5–7.5 cm i.d.) are recommended for faster flow rates. Best results are obtained if columns are fitted with column reservoirs to allow one-step pouring.
4. Allow maximum gravity flow rate. (Do not pump.)
5. Stop column flow rate once all the medium has gone through the column.
6. Elute with Affi-Prep protein A binding buffer (Bio-Rad Laboratories).
7. As the column elution progresses, two color bands (red and yellow) will develop. The red band is caused by the concentration of the tissue culture medium pH indicator, phenol red, as it is removed from the column. An adjacent yellowish band containing IgG and other proteins is observed ahead of the red band.
8. Collect both red and yellow bands to ensure good immunoglobulin recovery. The sample is now ready to be chromatographed on Affi-Prep protein A (or other columns).

---

*This centrifugation step is designed to remove any remaining particles and lipids that tend to hinder the ultrafiltration procedure (step 10). When large quantities of ascites render ultracentrifugation difficult, ultrafiltration can be performed directly as long as prefilters are used to avoid clogging of the 0.22 μm membrane filter. Also, the lipid removal step is not necessary as long as protein A chromatography is performed prior to hydroxylapatite chromatography as recommended in this chapter. Alternatively, ascites can be diluted 10-fold with loading buffer.

Index